HARD TIMES AND GREAT BLESSINGS

THE STORY OF MY LIFE

KENNETH F. WORTH

Outskirts Press, Inc.
Denver, Colorado

The opinions expressed in this manuscript are solely the opinions of the author and do not represent the opinions or thoughts of the publisher. The author represents and warrants that s/he either owns or has the legal right to publish all material in this book.

Hard Times and Great Blessings
The Story of My Life
All Rights Reserved.
Copyright © 2008 Kenneth F. Worth
V2.0

Cover Photo © 2008 JupiterImages Corporation. All rights reserved - used with permission.

This book may not be reproduced, transmitted, or stored in whole or in part by any means, including graphic, electronic, or mechanical without the express written consent of the publisher except in the case of brief quotations embodied in critical articles and reviews.

Outskirts Press, Inc.
http://www.outskirtspress.com

ISBN: 978-1-4327-2308-8

Outskirts Press and the "OP" logo are trademarks belonging to Outskirts Press, Inc.

PRINTED IN THE UNITED STATES OF AMERICA

TABLE OF CONTENTS

DEDICATION
PREFACE
CHAPTER 1 - ORPHANED 1
CHAPTER 2 - SAVING GRACE 13
CHAPTER 3 - GROWING UP 25
CHAPTER 4 - VIETNAM 39
CHAPTER 5 - CAREER 59
CHAPTER 6 - THE ARSENAL 73
CHAPTER 7 - RETIRED 95
CHAPTER 8 - TRIALS and BLESSINGS 101
EPILOGUE 111

DEDICATION

Dedicating this book was difficult. There are many people who have significantly impacted my life for the better. I could not pick only one person. There are two women who have had a life-changing impact on me. I will forever appreciate both of them. They are my mother-in-law Theresa and my wife Ruth.

My mother-in-law took me into her heart, and I'm sure prayed daily for me. She encouraged me and continually told me about the Lord. She literally would not give up on me. Without her prodding, I probably would not have found Jesus. I also would not have gone to college. My whole life would have been different—for the worse. She entered my life when I was deciding what path to travel. But for her, I would have taken the wrong road. Thank you, "Mom." I'll see you in heaven soon. Mom Beck died February 11, 1996, at 5:00 A.M. She is with Jesus.

My wife Ruth and I are "attached at the hip." We have been married for 48 years. Without her I'm useless. She is the love of my life. I met her in church after I met her parents. We went together for five years before we were married. Her influence on me and on my life choices has been indescribable. She loves the Lord, and she has loved me in spite of my problems.

Ruth and her mother were an indomitable team. They got me! Thank you, Ruth. I'll love you forever on earth and in heaven.

I would also like to thank Ruth for helping me remember many details from our lives. Thanks also to my daughter, Julia, and to Julia's husband, Rob, for their help with the editing and to my daughter Cheryl for permission to use her story "In Over My Head."

PREFACE

There is nothing more constant than change. I have seen this many times through sixty-eight years of life experiences, and it is still true! My life was and is full of change. Over the years as I have related some of my experiences at family gatherings and other places, I have been asked, "Why don't you write a book?" I didn't give it much thought. Recently, I wrote an article about my life for a support group publication. I received many favorable comments, and once again I was confronted with the question, "Why don't you write a book?"

I saw my life as nothing special, but many other people said they found my experiences to be interesting and a help to them. Some felt it gave them comfort and hope. I decided to do it. This book is the result. This is a true story. As a courtesy to other people involved in my story, I have changed some of the names.

If you are looking for an action-packed book, you are in the wrong place. This is my life. I hope you find it interesting. It has been a life full of hard times and great blessings, a life that I would not exchange with anyone. God gave me this life. I don't know why, but this I do know—with His help I will finish the journey.

CHAPTER 1
ORPHANED

BANG! I did not hear the shot nor the one that followed it sometime later that morning. I must have slept through it. BANG! This was the unwanted beginning of the rest of my life. I had just turned eleven years old. My older brother Carl and I were asleep in our small bedroom. Why did we not hear the shots? It didn't make any sense. We had become orphans that day. Our lives would be changed forever. The details will come later. We will start at the beginning.

It all started on August 20, 1939, the day I was born in Fitkin Hospital, Neptune, New Jersey. My older brother Carl had been born three years earlier in the same hospital. The old hospital is still there today, though it has undergone significant changes, including a new name (Jersey Shore University Medical Center).

I don't remember much about my early life or what we did as a family. I wish I did. My dad Lester was eight years older than my mom Nellie. I believe they had been married for about five years before I was born. We were not well off financially, but neither were we dirt-poor. Most people would say we were a happy family. Dad had retired due to a back injury. He could not do any heavy lifting. But he continued to labor as a house-wrecker when he could get the work. Mom was a homemaker before that became a popular word.

When Mom was younger she used to sing in church. But by the time I came on the scene she didn't go to church anymore. Dad didn't either. Mom did see to it that my brother and I went to Sunday school on a regular basis.

We lived in a very small house in Neptune City, New Jersey. Life in those days was relatively simple. My memories of us as a family are all good. We spent our time playing with what few friends we had. In those days playing outside was not a problem. Yes, life really was simple for a small boy, and things were going along well.

Some years later (my flawed memory says it was about August, 1945, when I was about six years old), we moved a short distance away to New Shrewsbury, New Jersey. We lived in a very small house with a store built across the front. My mom took care of running the store with Dad helping out when he could. We lived on Route #33 on a three and one-half acre farm at the bottom of a traffic circle. It was a small piece of land that was not operated as a working farm at the time. Route #33 was very busy with traffic, but it was a good location for the store. The first real memories that I have of my early life begin here.

While we lived in New Shrewsbury, Carl and I went to school at the Tinton Falls Schools. The school bus picked us up from the front of our store. The only thing noteworthy at school was that I had a crush on one of the teachers, Mrs. Dougherty. I remember that she was very kind to me and seemed to spend more time with me than with some of the others in the class. This was probably because I was shy. Like all such crushes, it didn't last long.

We had four homes on our property along with some small outbuildings, including a run-down chicken coop. One of my jobs around the farm was cleaning up the chicken coop. I had to do this every couple of days. I had to feed the chickens and gather the eggs every day. In fact, I ended up being the one that took care of all the animals on the farm. Fortunately, we didn't have many animals.

My dad had rented out three of the houses on our property, and we lived in the other one with the store. Dad had built all the homes, mainly from old wood and other building materials he had gleaned from houses he had helped to demolish. Life still was not bad. Not yet. We still didn't know that we didn't have much. We were a normal family and pretty much kept to ourselves. Mom and Dad did not socialize.

Dad had some hunting dogs he took out in the woods on hunting trips. He really enjoyed his hunting and took the dogs out whenever he could. I recall that they were outside dogs, so we could not play with them. My brother and I wished that Dad would get an inside dog that we could play with. Besides the dogs, we always had a few cats around. The cats lived outside also. As you might expect, living next to a busy highway we lost many cats to the traffic!

Family fun in those days was sitting or lying on the floor in the living room listening to our favorite radio programs like Jack Benny, The Shadow, The Lone Ranger, and many others. We would make it a family affair and follow the shows religiously. Then, around 1949, we got a black and white television set. It was one of the first in the area. What a tiny screen! When there was a program on, we would sit around and watch the microscopic picture. The TV did not broadcast all day, and there were only a few stations. It seems so silly now, but I remember watching in fascination as the test pattern displayed on the screen in between broadcast times.

I remember playing with our friends Jack and Chuck whose parents owned the Chapman lumberyard about a quarter of a mile down the road. Playing in the lumberyard was fun. We would run through the yard and then climb all over the stacks of lumber only to be chased off by the owner, Mr. Chapman. Playing on our farm was also fun because we had plenty of room to play and so many things to do.

Though we had a farm, we grew only some

small items for our own use. We grew corn and a few vegetables. I used to eat the tomatoes right off the vines. That is the way to eat tomatoes! But for my brother and I, the really important thing growing on the farm was a huge walnut tree that we used as a base when we played tag. We also would crack open the nuts and eat them. Like any boys our age, we found ways to have fun on the farm.

We also found ways to get in trouble. Another area we used to play in was the woods behind our rented homes. Jack and Chuck would come over from the lumber yard to play with us on the farm. I remember taking cigarettes from our store and smoking them in the woods behind the houses. Boy, did we get it when Mom finally figured it out and caught us! It was one of the few times that Mom really got mad at us. My dad smoked, and she was determined that we would not.

Dad was clearing a small field to plant some more corn. We used Dad's old truck to pull out the stumps. I believe it was a 1940 Ford that had been around the block more than a few times. Pulling stumps out with an old truck is not fun, but it surely beats digging them out by hand. Dad did as much of the work as he could, but my brother and I had to do a lot of the work because of Dad's bad back.

We used to think that Dad was a tough guy. He would tell us what good shape he was in and have us punch him in the stomach as hard as we could. He would have no reaction to the punches. Then he would laugh. We didn't think about his back problems, and he seemed to be able to do much of the work around the farm.

Sometimes in the afternoon Dad would take us for rides in his old truck. It was great fun when Dad would let me sit on his lap and steer the truck. Mom would always tell us the dangers of what we were doing, but we would do it anyway.

Life on the farm did have its hazards. One day Dad was trying to pound down a piece of metal that was sticking out from the end of a long pipe. I don't know what Dad was going to use the pipe for, but he was using a heavy mallet to pound down the piece that was sticking out. I can't remember why, but Carl was holding the other end of the pipe on his shoulder. Carl shifted the pipe over his head towards the other shoulder at the same time that Dad hit the pipe with the mallet. The pipe came down on Carl's head. I'm sure the bleeding looked worse than it was. That episode required a trip to the hospital and a few stitches. Once we knew Carl was okay we had a good laugh over his bald spot around the wound.

Then there was the time Carl and I were running around the yard playing tag. Carl jumped over the barbed wire fence Dad had put up. We had done this many times, but this time Carl judged incorrectly and landed in the fence. Once he was in the air he realized that he had jumped too soon, but it was too late and he could not pull his feet up far enough to clear the wire. That required another trip to the emergency room and a few more stitches.

I had my own share of visits to the hospital. I

HARD TIMES AND GREAT BLESSINGS

remember being there to have my tonsils taken out and that the nurse gave me ice cream to eat after the operation. On another occasion, I was running in the house. Mom told me not to do it, but I did not listen. I tripped and fell, going through the doorway to the living room. I didn't know there was a nail sticking up in the doorway. Dad had it on his list of things to fix. I fell and the nail went right through the soft tissue of my chin. We made yet another trip to the emergency room. Fortunately, it did not do any permanent damage. That was just part of being an active boy.

One day I fell down while running in the house and the sharp end of a lead pencil pierced the skin just above my right eye. The point broke off and a piece of lead had to be removed. I'm not sure we got all of it out. Sometimes I feel a slight bump over my right eye. I wonder if some of the lead is still in there.

We used to watch Dad cut off the chickens' heads. What a funny sight to see! Chickens ran around the yard with their heads cut off. Since we were next to a busy highway, sometimes the chickens would even make it to the road and get hit by passing cars. It's one of those "You have to see it to get it" kind of things!

Then there was Mr. Carter. He was the local driver for Abbots Ice Cream. He delivered to the New Shrewsbury area, and our store was on his route. He was very nice to us. We would stop whatever we were doing and watch him unload his ice cream products. Sometimes we would help carry them into our store. We would stand by his truck, and he would give us free ice cream. I didn't know it then, but eventually I would meet his son Gary and we would become close friends.

Even when I was very young, not everything was fun and games. My nights were especially scary. I was afraid of the dark. I tried to stay up as long as possible, but Mom would make me go to bed. I would lay in bed and think I saw things or heard noises in the closet. I bet you have had this experience too. The room was small and dark, and the closet was close to my bed. Though I got over this later in life, I still am uneasy in total darkness.

I remember going to Sunday school in a small Methodist church just a few miles away. We would stand at the top of the traffic circle and a church bus would pick us up every Sunday. It was a church that laid out the gospel in simple terms that I could understand, but I didn't want any of what they were preaching. Life was going good without it. We really did not want to go to Sunday school, but Mom made sure we did. She knew that this would help us later in life.

I had wanted a clock radio for some time, but we could not afford one. I had asked for one numerous times but to no avail. Then, on August 20, 1950, my eleventh birthday, I got it! Mom and Dad had gotten it at Shafto's Appliance store down the road. Actually, they gave it to me a couple of days before my birthday, which was very unusual. I liked it a lot and couldn't wait to set the alarm and play the radio. I didn't know at the time that it wasn't paid for and never would be. I didn't find out for years. All I knew was that I liked it and that I was happy. After I set the alarm, it would wake me up to music in the morning. I felt good and things were going along fine.

Then, two days after my birthday, it happened. My whole world came crashing down. **BANG! BANG!** Mercifully, my brother and I did not hear the shots. To this day, we don't know for sure exactly what happened. Though I am writing this some fifty-eight years later, I still have a problem talking or thinking about it. The easy life was over in seconds. The hard part began.

It was August 22, 1950. It was early morning. My brother Carl got up first and went looking for Mom because he wanted breakfast. Mom usually got up before us and normally had to wake us up. It was unusual for her not to be up now. Carl looked all over the house to find her. She was nowhere to be found. Instead, he found Dad lying on his back in bed. It was not a sight for a fourteen-year-old to see. We did not know it then, but Dad had been shot in the head with a 12-gauge shotgun. He had no head left. There were just pieces of skin and bone laying on what was left of his pillow.

Carl came and got me. We looked around again but could not find Mom. I went into the bedroom to see Dad. I shouldn't have. It was a terrible sight to see. We didn't know what to do, so we went to one of our rented houses where the Whites lived, and Mrs. White came down to our house. When she saw Dad, she took a nickel out of the cash register in the store and called the police.

I don't remember much else that happened after that. I do recall how the police talked to us and then got us out of the house. But it is fifty-eight years later, and I still see Dad lying there with no head. You don't heal easily from this kind of memory. Hard times come. Dad was forty-five years old and had three sisters and two brothers. Though this made the front page of the Asbury Park Press, my brother and I did not see any of it because all the details were kept from us.

The next thing I remember was being in Neptune City, New Jersey, in the home of my maternal grandparents Ike and Selena Newman. The police had called them and took us to their home, which was not that far from where we lived. I never really knew anyone on my father's side of the family. I'm sure we had seen them but I didn't remember them.

As I mentioned, my brother and I were never given the official version of what happened and why. All the details were withheld from us. We didn't know it, but the police had searched our house and found my mother at the bottom of the cellar stairs. She had been shot in the stomach with the same 12-gauge shotgun. It was Dad's shotgun. Fortunately, we had not seen Mom's body. Mom was 37 years old and had one sister and four brothers.

HARD TIMES AND GREAT BLESSINGS

Years later we obtained copies of the original newspaper articles from the Asbury Park Press. We found out that the first assistant prosecutor had investigated and called it murder/suicide. We never have found out for sure what happened, but it appears that Mom shot Dad and then herself. Murder/suicide has been hard to accept. I have often wondered, will I see my mom and dad in heaven? I intend to be there and I will look for them.

The funeral was "closed casket" and was held at the Clayton Funeral Home in Adelphia, New Jersey. My parents were buried close to our home in Monmouth Memorial Park on Route #33 in New Shrewsbury, New Jersey. There was a fairly large crowd at the funeral, and, though no one said much to my brother and me, we were the talk of the town. We were orphans. It began to sink in. Mom and Dad were not coming back! What would we do without our parents? Where would we live?

The next thing I remember is a meeting in my grandparents' house. I'll never forget it. Carl and I were told to go to bed, but we were in the bedroom listening at the door. The meeting was to decide who we would go and live with. Members of both sides of my family were there. I didn't know many of them. As we listened through the door, we could hear them talking.

Some said they would take us for the money the state would pay them. Others did not want us at all. This was hard to listen to, and I still can hear it. Eventually, Grandpa Ike took control of the meeting and emphatically said he would keep us. He did! He would not allow us to go to a family that just wanted us for the money. Some people there were unhappy, but it was decided. We would stay with my grandparents. For Carl and I, this decision would shape our future. But at the time, we did not understand the potential impact of this decision. We just were concerned about where we would live and what we would do now.

My grandfather was in his sixties when we came to live with him. He was a carpenter. I will always be grateful to my grandparents for taking us in to live with them. Only later—many years later—did I realize what effect this would have on my life. I did not realize it at the time, but there was another carpenter working behind the scenes in my life. A carpenter from Nazareth.

My grandparents were a godsend. They made sure we went to church every Sunday. They did the best they could to raise us properly. But the generation gap was huge. In time, I became rebellious. Probably because he was older and also because of what he had been through, my brother Carl became even more rebellious than me. We did not realize it then but many years of hard times were ahead for both of us. Mercifully, there were also to be many times of great blessings. Such was my life up to age eleven.

Yet life moved on.

CHAPTER 2
SAVING GRACE

The next part of my life was one of hard times. Carl and I were orphans let loose in the world without any preparation. We were mad that Mom and Dad were dead and that this situation was thrust on us. One second I was a boy with no real major concerns, and the next second I was expected to be a man. It does not work that way. It seemed like the weight of the world was on my shoulders.

My brother Carl was descending the same slippery slope as I was but at a much faster rate of speed. Neither of us adapted well to living with my grandparents. However, though I was feeling sorry for myself, I adjusted much better than Carl did. Yet neither of us knew what to do. We both did not want to be there, but we had no other options. I wanted my mother. It wasn't our grandparents' fault. They treated us well. In fact, they treated us much better than we treated them. But they had a task ahead that was just too big. The generation gap and the things we had just been through had impacted our lives in a way that was beyond our grandparents' ability to overcome.

You cannot understand how either of us felt unless you have been through a similar situation. It was not fair! Why did it happen to us? Why did God allow it? We had a lot of questions but no answers. We probably needed to seek God's help, but we were too mad at Him for letting this happen.

Looking back now, I can see that living with my grandparents was a great blessing. But at the time it didn't seem so to us. Grandpa tried to include us in as many things as he could and took us with him whenever possible. I remember how he took us along to the dealer when he bought another Pontiac. He liked those cars, and so did I. They took us to the auction, but we would peel off as soon as we could and walk around on our own. Grandpa would also take us with him into his combination garage and shop when he was working on something, but this was not often.

We went crabbing and clamming with them. Grandma loved to go crabbing. She would sit near the water along the pier for hours where she would drop in her "crab box" with the fish head in it as bait. The water level had to be just the right depth, not too deep or too shallow. Grandma would do her crocheting while she was crabbing. Grandpa loved to go clam digging. He would go out on the sandy beaches and with his bare feet would locate the clams and dig them up. Of course, Carl and I were bored stiff during these outings. There wasn't much for us to do with our grandparents. We just didn't like the same things and places that they liked.

Carl began to get in trouble frequently. He wanted to be on his own, and he took action by running away from home repeatedly. He loved Florida and kept going back there. I can remember the calls my grandparents received from the police in Florida when they would find Carl.

While we lived in Neptune City with my grandparents Carl and I started hanging around with the wrong crowd. We would walk the streets, especially when it was dark, and we were constantly getting in trouble. It was over petty kinds of wrongdoing, but we were consistent about finding one way or another to keep ourselves in trouble. We were a real burden on my grandparents who had a difficult time taking care of us and trying to raise us properly. They were not equipped for raising two more kids, especially considering their ages and the kinds of problems we had. Years passed, but we did not get any better.

I remember walking the streets at night near our grandparents' home. It seemed that we were pushing the envelope and trying to find ways to make problems for ourselves. I especially remember my grandfather walking the streets behind us as we stayed just far enough ahead of him so that he could not catch up. It was quite a sight, Grandpa following us, calling our names, while we went block after block, throwing rocks along the way to break out the street lights. After our escapades, we really got it when we finally went home. We would be grounded, but we didn't care and would do it all over again as soon as we were allowed to go out. I am sorry I put so much grief and pressure on my grandparents. They did not deserve to be treated like that. They are with the Lord now enjoying their rewards.

Remember Mr. Carter the ice cream man who used to deliver ice cream to our store? He lived in Neptune City. When we moved to my grandparents' house in Neptune City, I met his son Gary, and we became close friends. We went to school together.

I remember that my grandmother used to make me a ham sandwich almost every day for lunch, and Gary's mother would make him peanut butter and jelly sandwiches. I liked peanut butter and jelly better than ham. Gary liked ham better than peanut butter and jelly. We used to swap sandwiches almost every day. We hung out together. Neither of us was very popular in school, but we got along very well together.

One day Gary and I were walking the streets not too far from where we lived. We came to a field that was overgrown with brush and surrounded by houses. Though we were just fooling around, we started a fire that quickly got out of hand. There was no reason for starting a fire but we did. We left quickly and watched from a distance. We did a good job of clearing the field. The police and two fire trucks came to put out the fire. Fortunately, there was no property damage, and no one was hurt. We didn't realize the magnitude of what we had done.

A few of us, usually three or four at a time, would skip school and go down to the boardwalk in Asbury Park. We would walk the boardwalk and the streets nearby for hours. Sometimes we would go to the beach or ride the rides in the amusement area. Sometimes we would go to the other nearby town's boardwalks or beaches, but we liked Asbury Park the best. The police would try to catch us, but we knew all the best hiding places in the boardwalk area. So we never did get caught.

Our group was made up of my brother Carl and Charlie who shared informal leadership. With us sometimes was George Jr. Another boy, John, was almost always with us. Then there was me. Carl used to try to get me to stay behind but I usually tagged along anyway. Carl was three years older than me, and that was enough for him to want his little brother not to hang around.

I remember how my friend Gary used to have a fourteen foot row boat with a five horsepower Johnson outboard motor. We would ride in it quite often. We would take it out in the ocean to fish for fluke. We would barely make it out of the inlet and into open water because the small motor could scarcely overcome the current. Somehow we usually made it. Sometimes the Coast Guard would catch us going out and would make us go back, but most of the time they were not around. The waves were sometimes too high, and we couldn't make it out of the inlet. It was fun but, as usual, we did not understand the danger in what we were doing.

Later, Gary got a fast speed boat. We had no problem getting out into the ocean with it, but it did sway a lot in the larger waves. When we were coming in one day to dock the boat, I reached out to grab hold of the rusty metal pole sticking out of the water so I could slow the boat down. I judged wrong and caught my hand between the boat and the pole. It really hurt. There was a "V" cut in my palm with what looked like chords sticking out of it. I washed it off with the dirty salt water and pushed the chords inside the wound. Then I got a band aid out of the first aid kit and put it on the wound. I was lucky. It healed up on its own over time and today I can hardly see the scar.

In the winter, we would stand at the top of a wooded hill and lob snowballs at passing cars and trucks. Occasionally, someone would stop and start chasing after us, but we knew how to get away quickly.

One summer while at the auction we met Roberto, a former golden gloves boxer. Roberto liked to hang around the auction. One day we took a ride with him in his car. Roberto's ride included spinning his tires through the turf around two greens on a nearby golf course. In time, we also discovered that he was very good at driving and had a reputation for spinning around in the snow when it was slippery enough.

One day as we were roaming the streets, we decided to take our misadventures to the next level

HARD TIMES AND GREAT BLESSINGS

and do something new. It was Saturday, and there was a factory nearby that appeared empty. We saw our opportunity when we found a window that was not locked, and we went inside to look around. We did not cause any real damage, but we did throw some stuff around and took a few dollars from an open desk drawer. We left the factory and followed the railroad tracks for a while.

We found other amusements the rest of the day. We came upon an old, run down, vacant house. The attic was loaded with pigeons, but the rest of the house was empty. One of our group, John, kept pigeons in a cage on the roof of his house. We decided we would come back later and take some pigeons to his house. But it didn't work out and we never did go back. We went back to following the tracks. We stopped to roll rocks down a hill, trying to land them on the tracks so that we could see them crushed by the trains. We had often placed pennies on the tracks to see the trains flatten them out. Again, we didn't realize the danger in what we were doing.

Our spree came to an end when we saw the flashing lights on a police car. This time they caught us. We got a ride to the police station and were interviewed. The police contacted our parents (grandparents in my case). As a result of our actions that day, one of our group, Charlie, who already had quite a criminal record and was well known by the police in Neptune, ended up in reform school. The rest of us were put on an informal probation.

KENNETH F. WORTH

Throughout this period, I continued to have some connection with the church. But it was only the thinnest of links. We used to go to the Full Gospel Assemblies of God church in Neptune, New Jersey. The pastor, Rev. Matheson, had started the church in a tent and ultimately pastored that same church for about fifty years. The church has since moved to another location in Wall Township. My grandparents made sure that we went to Sunday school every Sunday morning. However, we would sneak out of Sunday school and church whenever we could and go down to the corner grocery store.

The store was owned by one of my cousins, Jason Myers. We would take our Sunday school money and instead of putting it in the offering we would spend it at the store. We liked going to the store. Jason made the biggest ice cream cones in the area. One day he weighed the ice cream he put on each cone and found out he was charging less per cone than he was actually paying for the ice cream. That was the end of his big cones.

My grandparents would often find out that we went down to the store instead of going to church. We would get in trouble, but we would go back again the next Sunday. Actually, we were more afraid of the Sunday school superintendent than we were of my grandparents. He would chew us out when he found out what we were doing, and he had a military way of dealing with us.

Sundays spent at the store did not improve my character. As my brother and I grew into our teenage years, we would take cigarettes from Jason's store. I would stuff them in a zippered pocket on my leather jacket. We would also take empty soda bottles from the back outside of Jason's store and take them around front and turn in each bottle for the two cent deposit. I was going through a stage in which I thought I was cool. I wore a black leather motorcycle jacket with enough zippered pockets on it for ten people. I used to go to Jason's house often, and his mother would heat up something for me to eat. I was not a good kid. I was not someone I'd want my children to emulate.

My grandparents took us to church at Full Gospel Church on Sunday mornings, and we went with them to a Pentecostal Church in Belmar on Sunday nights. The Belmar church was a lively place. People were speaking in tongues and dancing in the aisles. Carl and I felt uneasy there, and we did not want to go to any church, but we had to go with my grandparents. It was not optional. My grandparents were tough on us, but now, looking back, I am glad they were.

They say boys will be boys. They need good physical outlets. We found our fun on the street. One of the things we used to do is "ride the bus." In the snow, we would hang onto the bumper of a moving bus or car and skate up the street on our shoes. The snow had to be wet and slippery for a good ride. The buses and cars would slow down to go up a hill. We would either grab onto the bumpers or offer them a push if they needed it. Then we would grab onto the bumpers. Many times they would make us get off. For us, it was all part of the challenge. The trick was getting on the bumper without the driver knowing about it. We got pretty good at it. "Riding the bus" was fun, but, as usual, we did not realize the danger we were in.

In 1952, when I was thirteen, we moved to West Belmar, New Jersey. I attended and completed Central Grammar School in Glendola. When I look back, I remember Frank the bully. He always used to give me and some others a hard time. He used to chase us around until one day I had enough and got mad. I stood up to him and ended up chasing him. I had no more trouble with Frank after that. At age fourteen, I started attending Manasquan High School in Manasquan, New Jersey. I did not know it, but I was about to have a major life change. It would be the most significant thing that ever happened to me.

Meanwhile, Carl turned eighteen and was living on his own. That put me on my own too. We were no longer a team, and though we had a special bond that few have, we would grow apart. Carl kept getting in trouble, but he had a loving spirit. There was something special about Carl that people were attracted to. Everyone liked Carl.

At church I had met Sister Beck through her husband Fred who was my Sunday school teacher. She knew of our situation and took an interest in Carl and me. There was something different about Sister Beck. She would make it a point to talk to me

HARD TIMES AND GREAT BLESSINGS

and make me feel special.

Sister Beck stayed on my case for what felt like years, telling me about Jesus. She was always talking about Jesus. Always Jesus, Jesus, Jesus. I was tired of hearing about Him. I did, however, know about Him from years of going to Sunday school and church. I knew inside that I was a sinner and needed to be saved, but I had resisted so long that I had no intention of doing any different on this particular Sunday. However, this Sunday church would be different. It started the same but somehow I knew that it was definitely going to end differently. It was May 22, 1955. I was fifteen years old.

Pastor Matheson had preached his sermon on salvation. The church service was over, but here came Sister Beck straight for me! I could not get away. I resisted her prodding for some time, but I could not hold her off. This time she brought help. I could feel it. The Holy Spirit was there, and He was not taking "No" for an answer. Much to my surprise, I was ready. I went to the altar and, with Sister Beck at my side, asked for forgiveness and salvation. I accepted Jesus as my personal savior that day. This was the singular, most significant thing I've ever done. My name is written in the book of life.

Thank you, Jesus!

CHAPTER 3
GROWING UP

Now that I had accepted the Lord, I expected that everything would go along perfectly and I would be constantly happy. After all, I was a child of God and a genuine Christian. I was ready for that continual happiness—really ready. However, I found out that this is not the way it actually works. We have to live in this world and are impacted with the same good and bad things that happen to everybody else. I found out that God never said He would keep us from every problem situation. My advantage, which I did not fully realize, and His promise to me was that He would go through every situation, every problem, and every part of my life with me. I would discover that was enough.

During the winter months my grandparents would go to Florida for about three months. They enjoyed Florida and did not like the cold weather in New Jersey during the winter. While they lived in Florida, I would go live with various relatives.

The first year I lived with my uncle Ben Walters

and his wife Marie in Neptune City. Ben had been a gardener for many years and was kept busy in the summer months but had free time during the winter. Ben and Marie had three children, Joel, Sarah, and Tim. I became good friends with Tim.

When living with my grandparents in West Belmar, I went to Manasquan High School. I was happy there. I liked going to that school a lot. I made some friends there. But when I lived with the Walters, I had to begin going to Neptune High School. I found that I did not fit in there. I didn't know anyone, and all my friends were at Manasquan.

After a year of going to Neptune High, I tried something different. And it worked. Every morning I would ride my bike from Uncle Ben's house in Neptune City to the bus stop in West Belmar where the bus to Manasquan High was parked and near where I lived with my grandparents. I would take the bus going to Manasquan High and I would attend my regular school. No one knew that I shouldn't have been there. I would ride my bike every winter day over this ten-mile round trip route.

Eventually, the Manasquan bus driver figured out what I was doing because I was early to the bus stop every day and because I had to leave my bike there in plain sight. He never did turn me in. In fact, he told me to put my bike in the garage area where it would not be stolen.

Sometimes while riding my bike to catch the school bus, I would "race" cars across the Shark

HARD TIMES AND GREAT BLESSINGS

River Bridge on the way to Neptune City. I had a three speed bike and could go extremely fast. One day I was riding my bike home from school as fast as I could. Suddenly, when I turned a familiar corner, I unexpectedly hit some sand on the road causing the rear tire to slip out from under me. I went down, landing on my left leg and skidding along the road for about ten feet. My pant leg ripped through, and my leg was scraped so much that it took off some of the skin. It hurt, but it had more like a stinging sensation. The bike was scraped up a little but was operationally okay. My leg took quite a while to heal, and I did not tell my grandparents the magnitude of the wound. It seemed like I was always getting scraped up or otherwise wounded.

Before Carl turned twenty-one, he decided to take out his inheritance. My parents had left a small estate from the sale of our farm. It was a very small inheritance, but it was enough that it would have helped toward going to college. But Carl was not interested in college. He wanted the cash now even though everyone advised him to leave it in savings for his college education. However, Carl did not take their advice.

He made a deal with Mr. Travis, our estate lawyer, who agreed to pay him a percentage of the value of the inheritance. In exchange, when Carl turned twenty-one, his actual estate payout would go to Mr. Travis. What Mr. Travis agreed to pay right away was not a lot of money, but it was enough for Carl to buy a shiny new 1957 Chevy convertible. It was a beautiful car, white outside with a bright red interior. It was one of the nicest cars made that year. It was a hot car—so hot and so fast that Carl received a ticket on the New Jersey Parkway for going over 110 miles per hour. Was a new car worth it? Carl had his pleasure in the short term, but he never did go to college. This had an adverse impact on his life in the future. I elected to leave my estate money in savings. This ended up being a good decision.

I used to walk to the auction from my grandparents' house on Friday, Saturday, and sometimes Sunday nights. This was a small auction complex in some rather old buildings, but it had quite a bit of goods for sale. The auctioneer was located at one end of the largest building. I worked at the auction for Bob, an auctioneer who each week auctioned off all kinds of things from the back of his large truck. He sold everything from knick-knacks to small appliances. I would work there and then spend hours walking around.

That local auction was the site of a lot of activities. I remember how I used to get submarine sandwiches from a Sorrento's Subs stand at the auction for $1.00 each. They were the best subs I ever ate. They do not make them like that anymore. Not all of my activities around the auction were so innocent, particularly before I became a Christian. The auction was less than a mile away from where I lived with my grandparents in West Belmar, so Carl and I would often walk the distance. On the way, we

AND GREAT BLESSINGS

...ratch the side of cars with a key
...compartments of cars that were

...age, I could not wait to get my
...ps I should say I could not wait
...w to me" car. Over the years I
...om a lot of places, including a
...area on the highway, a used car
...n individual and new and used
...started to drive, I have owned

...rd sedan. That was my first car.
...dge Coronet with fluid drive.
- A dark green 1949 Mercury Coupe. A cool car!
- A black 1950 Ford sedan.
- A white 1953 Chevy Bel Air sedan.
- A light blue 1954 Chevy Bel Air convertible.
- A light blue 1960 Ford Fairlane 500.
- A yellow 1966 Ford Mustang.
- A burgundy 1969 Dodge Coronet with black roof.
- A cream 1968 Ford Country Squire station wagon.
- A light brown 1977 Pontiac Grand Prix.
- A white 1983 Cavalier. Bought over the phone.
- A burgundy 1987 Ford Taurus.
- A burgundy 1995 Ford Taurus.
- A harvest gold 2001 Ford Taurus, which I still have.

KENNETH F. WORTH

There are interesting stories to tell about some of the cars, and I'll tell them as we go along. I was surprised when I went back and counted how many cars I have owned and how many stories there are for specific cars.

As soon as I was old enough, I got my driver's license and started looking for my first car. I found it on a lot on highway #35 in Manasquan. It was sitting there with a "For Sale" sign in the window. I called the number on the sign and arranged for a test drive. The car had been around the block a few times, but it appeared to be working good and the motor sounded great. Also, and most importantly, it was within my limited budget. It was a green 1948 Ford with a high roof line. It looked like a turtle! I had to be careful going fast around corners because it was so top-heavy.

Once I got my Ford, I raced any car that would take me on. We would race up highway #35 to the Manasquan circle. I couldn't take off as fast as some cars, but I would keep the gas peddle to the floor until I won or ran out of room. I didn't lose many races. Many times I came up on the Manasquan circle at such a high rate of speed that I just about did not make it through the circle because I was going too fast to make the turn.

When racing I would shift from first to second gear at 50 mph and into third at 80 mph. My cousin, Tim Walters, could shift without engaging the clutch. This took some skill, and I never could get the hang of it. Not surprisingly, even though my

HARD TIMES AND GREAT BLESSINGS

Ford ran well for a while, it finally started to smoke and run bad. As you will see, that would be the story of my life.

My third car was a dark green 1949 Mercury. It was a cool looking car with skirts and a tiny window in the back. It also looked like a turtle and was top-heavy. I bought it from a gas station, and it was running fine at the time. It was a hot car and could really move. However, it wasn't long until it started to go. I had thought it was in good shape, but I was no mechanic. The gas station I bought it from had apparently fixed it up to run well for a short time, but that time was over.

While the Mercury was still running well, I used to roll the windows down, turn the radio on loud and drive slowly through the shore towns. This is what we did in those days. We also used to use this car to sneak some boys into the drive-in movies. They would squeeze into the trunk and get out inside the movie lot.

One time I remember being in Manasquan and the car got stuck in reverse. I did not have the money to get it fixed or towed, so I drove it backwards for about fifteen miles through the Manasquan circle and to the Becks' house in Wall Township. Fred Beck was a skilled mechanic. He knew that I did not have the money to get the car fixed, so he took the transmission apart, fixed it, and put it back together. I never had any trouble with the transmission after that, although when I would step hard on the gas two large circles of smoke would pour out of the twin exhaust.

Over time the car started to give me trouble. Everything started to go, and it finally died and was not worth repairing. I decided to take it to the junk yard. Tim borrowed a truck from work and he pushed me to the junk yard. When we came to the yard, he backed off, and I coasted in. The owner saw us come in and thought we drove in normally. He asked if the car still ran. I told him yes and gave him the bill of sale. He did not check the car and gave me cash for it. We quickly left and didn't look back. He didn't know that the motor had been stripped clean. The generator, spark plugs, wires, distributor, battery and anything else that would come out were already long gone.

From 1955 to 1962 I worked at the Acme Markets in Belmar and Elberon. Other than the auction, this was my first real job. George Snyder Sr., a district manager for Acme and a member of our church, got me the job. His son George Jr., was a "member" of our street-roaming group.

We continued to attend the Full Gospel Church on Sunday mornings, but we stopped attending the Pentecostal church on Sunday evenings in Belmar. Apparently, my grandfather had a difference of opinion with the pastor. We were active in the Neptune church. I helped my grandfather rebuild a new back wall on the platform. It was all paneling and had hidden doors for the baptismal area. It got rave reviews from the congregation.

I remember one year one of the board members,

HARD TIMES AND GREAT BLESSINGS

Sam Mason, was in a Christmas play. As he was saying his part, he leaned against the hidden door and—you guessed it—suddenly disappeared from view. Then he came back in and said, "I'm back," as the crowd broke into laughter. After all, Grandpa was an excellent carpenter. And the doors were meant to be invisible.

Years later, after my wife and I were married, my brother-in-law Bill and I took over the boys club at the Full Gospel Church. It was part of an Assemblies of God program called the Royal Rangers. At first, only a few boys attended, all of whom went to the church. Bill and I went out on the streets and brought in any boys who would come. The club grew to over fifty.

We began to drive a church school bus along an hour and a half shore route to pick up many of the boys. I remember Chris Stevens, a twelve year old who was in a wheelchair. Bill and I used to carry him on and off the bus. This was difficult as I was wearing a metal brace for a bad back at the time, but Chris wanted to go, so we made sure he got there.

We took the boys on camping trips and other outings and even to Washington, D.C., to the Smithsonian Institute. That is an interesting story. We contacted Fort Meade, Virginia, about our Royal Rangers outpost staying in the barracks. We found out that certain groups were allowed to stay overnight in the barracks but only those who were written in the regulations by name.

There was an approval process for non-listed

groups, but they had to be a group of underprivileged kids to stand a chance of being approved. A key to having the request approved was fulfilling the requirement that the police sign a statement that the group was made up of underprivileged children. We went to the police station and began to tell the officer the names of our boys and where they lived. After we mentioned only a few, the officer quickly signed the letter. We submitted our request, which was approved, and then we took the boys to Washington, D.C.

While we were in the Smithsonian, some of our boys slipped away alone to go to the men's room. We had told the boys that they could not go to the restrooms alone. When we realized they were missing, Bill and I went into the men's room to get our boys out. It was not a minute too soon. There were two older boys hanging around the men's room, and it was obvious that our boys could have been in trouble. Our boys knew the rules, and they had broken them. So we packed up and left early for home.

While we were going home we ran into another situation. We were in a big blue church school bus. We were on a four lane road with an island in the middle. There was moderate traffic, and it was getting dark. Bill was driving. We needed gas, so he turned left to cross over the other two lanes to a gas station on the other side. All of a sudden, the bus quit—leaving us stranded broadside right across the two oncoming lanes. We could see the traffic coming at us. Apparently, the battery had died. To make matters worse, all the lights on the bus went off. The bus wouldn't start. We had a serious and dangerous situation and not much time to react.

With no time to get all the boys off, I ran up the road frantically waving my arms. God is good. There was a big 18-wheeler coming straight for us. The driver saw us and reacted quickly by maneuvering the truck across the road to block the traffic. We were able to get all the boys off, and we had enough people to push the bus off the road and into a gas station lot. What could have been a tragedy was averted. Everyone got home safely.

In 1954 I was still living with my grandparents. I was in Fred Beck's Sunday school class. He was an excellent teacher, and he ruled his class. I remember when I was fooling around in his class, he had this way of twisting my ear. It worked. I liked him a lot and behaved pretty well in his class.

His class had some rough boys in it, but Fred taught them the Bible in such a way that they actually were interested and learned things that would help them throughout their lives. I guess he felt sorry for me, and he invited me to his house to visit and eat. That is where I really got to know Sister Beck. She became like a mother to me.

I got in the habit of going to the Becks' house. At first, I went to see my Sunday school teacher Fred. But while I was there I got to know Sister Beck, and soon I was going to see her. She began to feed me. Soon I was a regular. Like my grandma,

Sister Beck was an excellent cook. But I didn't eat much at my grandparents. They were light eaters. But I ate quite a bit at the Becks'. I especially liked her spicy hot pot roast and gravy. It was delicious! At that stage of my life, I could eat all day and not gain any weight. Oh, that it was the same today! Sister Beck took me under her wing and into her heart.

It was there that I got to know the Becks' daughter Ruth and their two sons Bob and Bill. At first I didn't pay any attention to them, but over time I starting noticing Ruth. Soon I was coming to see her and not Fred or his wife Theresa. I did not know it at the time, but Ruth had liked me since she was in the seventh grade. Neither Ruth nor I dated anyone else before. Things progressed, and after a while we were officially going together.

The Becks set up some real strict rules for Ruth and me. We did not dare break them. As I look back, I understand that we had been going together long enough that her family considered such restrictions necessary. However, at the time, we didn't like or see the need for the restrictions. We had to be in by 10 P.M. and usually could not be alone. Being in the car alone was a no-no except for going directly to or from church. The Becks even knew just how long the trip took. There wasn't much we could do. Movies, bowling, and rollerskating were all out. Bummer! Through it all, I think we ended up okay, and all the restrictions probably helped.

HARD TIMES AND GREAT BLESSINGS

I remember the first time we kissed. It was 1957 and Ruth was a freshman in Manasquan High School. As I was getting ready to leave the Becks' house that evening, Ruth and I were saying goodbye as we had done numerous times before. However, this night would be different. As we both stood there nervously talking, I did it. I kissed her. Wow! We had waited so long for this moment. Bells rang and fireworks went off! It was worth the wait.

In 1958, I started attending Monmouth College (now Monmouth University). It was a miracle that I was accepted by the college. My grade point average (GPA) was not very good because I got mostly C's with an occasional B and a smattering of D's. I had no interest in college and was not concerned about my GPA at the time. I'm not making light of my college education because I did see the light and I did do the work to graduate. I just did not have the right attitude going in and just made it through.

Ruth and I went together for five years. I asked her to marry me on October 15, 1959. Of course I asked her parents for their blessing first. Then that night I placed the ring on her finger—we were engaged. Our plans were to get married after Ruth's graduation from high school in June and her birthday in July, 1960. She would be eighteen and I would be twenty-one in August. We knew we were compatible after going together for five years.

We had the usual concerns that every couple has when planning their wedding that everything would be perfect. We also were concerned about "protecting" our car as it was customary in our area to "enhance" the appearance of the newlyweds' car for their wedding day the night before by soaping up the windows, draping toilet paper all over the car and of course hanging cans off the rear bumper. Mr. Jensen, the produce manager in the Acme Market where I worked, was a lifesaver because he let us park our car on his lot the night before we got married. Fortunately our car was not touched.

We were married by Rev. Matheson in the Full Gospel Church on September 3, 1960. It was a beautiful wedding. Life seemed to be going well, but hard times were on the way again.

CHAPTER 4
VIETNAM

Ruth and I were finally married, and it was great. We had waited a long time for this. It had been five years since we started going together. Now we were looking for a new life together—a good life without some of the hardships we were used to going through.

Unfortunately, we started off on the wrong foot. Being naive about such things, we had not made reservations for our honeymoon night and had to drive for what seemed like forever until we found a motel with a vacancy. We had not considered that it was Labor Day weekend and that the motels would be booked solid. Finally, we found a vacancy and we ended up staying in an older motel which was just off one of the New Jersey Turnpike exits. I don't remember the name of the motel, but it has since been torn down. Our honeymoon was definitely not starting out as an example of what honeymoons were supposed to be like. We could only hope this was not a sign of things to come.

The next morning we headed toward Williamsburg, Virginia, and our designated honeymoon site, the Village of Williamsburg. We had driven from New Jersey to Virginia in our 1950 Ford. We had put four new tires on it for the trip. The car had been running well and we were not expecting any problems. However, we had not gone very far when the car started overheating. We stopped at a gas station and added some water to the radiator and decided to continue to Virginia. The car overheated again and we filled it up with water again. This cycle continued all the way to Williamsburg.

We had originally expected to stay at Williamsburg about a week, but we ended up staying only one day. The car was running so badly that we decided to end our honeymoon and make a run for it home to our apartment. We had some interesting experiences already on our honeymoon that would make good stories to tell our kids some day.

The next day we started home, but the heat-up and fill-up cycle got worse. We didn't dare shut off the engine for fear that it would not start again. Finally, the car just quit. Fortunately, it was right in front of a gas station. We were in Golansville, Virginia, far from home and stuck with a broken down car.

After looking at the car, the gas station owner told us that the engine block had cracked and running it in that condition had made it worse. It could not be fixed without a significant infusion of cash. We found a simple solution. The owner gave us $30.00 cash for the car, and we gave him the keys. The deed was done, and we were without a car. We owed more for the new tires that we had put on for the trip than we had gotten paid for the car. We told the owner that we would send him the bill of sale. How would we get home? How would we get around without a car?

But this saga was not over yet. We still had to get home. We put what we could of our stuff in one suitcase and one large box and left the rest in the car. We got a ride over to a nearby country store where we bought bus tickets home. We were told that because of the heavy traffic on the highway the bus would not stop for us unless the driver saw us in time. We had to stand on the edge of the highway while the traffic sped by about a foot or so in front of us. Finally the bus stopped and picked us up. On the bus, it was standing room only. We stood in the aisle with our box and suitcase at our feet for most of the trip to New Jersey. Ruth had called one of her best friends, Marie Turner, to pick us up at a bus stop and take us to our apartment. What a way to start off our married life!

We arrived home from our unusual honeymoon to our ground floor apartment in Ocean Grove, New Jersey. This was the first place we lived together as husband and wife. It was an old house. The leaky windows did double duty, allowing the wind to blow in and allowing massive amounts of heat to blow out. The thermostat for the two apartments in the building was in our apartment. Needless to say, adjusting the heat properly so everyone was happy and reasonably comfortable was almost impossible.

The cost of heating the apartment in Ocean Grove was very high, especially when added to the rent and electric. Also, it was inconvenient to stay in Ocean Grove because it was a controlled area and you could not park your car in the Grove on Sundays. You had to park outside and walk in to your house. Depending on where you lived in the Grove, you could walk many blocks. All these things led us to look for another apartment. In those days an apartment complex was very rare.

It took some looking, but we found an upstairs apartment in Bradley Beach. It belonged to our estate lawyer, Mr. Travis. We rented it and made a deal with the lawyer to fix the place up in lieu of the first month's $85.00 rent. With Fred Beck's help, we did just that. New paint, new shelves in the kitchen, and a lot of cleaning gave the place a good face lift resulting in an apartment substantially better than when we moved in.

Since our car had broken down on our honeymoon, we were without transportation. We desperately needed another car but could not afford one. In the process of looking for a car, we stopped in Belmar at the Matt Fox Ford dealership. Ruth and I wanted to buy a new car, but we only had $25.00 between us. The rest of our honeymoon money was gone. We were very disappointed that the salesman and manager would not sell us a new car with only $25.00 down. We were even willing to take a basic car with no extras.

HARD TIMES AND GREAT BLESSINGS

Once again, a blessing came. It just so happened that Matt Fox himself was at the dealership while we were there. He was a well-known local golf pro who happened to own a Ford dealership. He apparently heard our story, felt sorry for us, and personally approved us for buying a new 1960 Ford Fairlane with only $25.00 down and the rest financed. *This car cost almost $2,000.00!*

We had that car for six years, and it was an excellent car. One funny thing though was that Ruth never drove the car for the entire six years we had it. It was a stick shift, which she did not know how to drive. However, the car was definitely a godsend.

In June 1963, I graduated from Monmouth College (now Monmouth University), Long Branch, New Jersey, with a BS degree in Business Administration with a major in accounting. I had started at Monmouth College in 1958, about two years before Ruth and I were married. That is a story in itself. I never intended to go to college. I didn't know what I was going to do with my life, and to be honest I didn't care much. This was not a priority or something that I thought about much. But that was about to change.

Remember Sister Beck? She was now "Mom" Beck, my mother-in-law. Even before Ruth and I were married, she was on my case about going to college. She wouldn't let up. She convinced me. Because of her persistence, I applied. Miraculously, I was accepted by Monmouth College. I would discover that this was another of God's blessings.

KENNETH F. WORTH

While I was going to college, I got a job as an auditor for the state of New Jersey. This was a very interesting job which required a lot of working in the field. My most interesting assignment was auditing the horse racing tracks in the state. It was fun to watch the horses practice and race and to verify that the winning tickets were valid. Vern was a senior auditor there, and I learned a lot about auditing from him in a short time frame. He was willing to pass on his experience and helped me grow into the job.

In August, 1963, I was 24 years old. I had just graduated from Monmouth College, and I was still working for the State Auditor. One day as I opened the mail, I saw what no young man wanted to see in 1963—a draft notice. It informed me that I had been drafted into the Army for two years. I hadn't given much thought to the future, and I had certainly given none to going into the Army for two or three years. I was still working for the State Auditor in New Jersey at the time and had planned to use this experience to advance in the financial management field. I was stunned. Where did this come from? Why me? Why now when everything looked so good?

When the Auditors Office found out that I had been drafted, they suggested that I join the National Guard before my draft date. Then I would only have weekend meetings and not have to be in the Army full time and possibly leave my wife. I just had to do it before my draft date. I didn't believe this

HARD TIMES AND GREAT BLESSINGS

option was the proper thing to do. Though I did not want to go into the Army, I also did not want to shirk my duty. Instead of joining the Guard, I enlisted in the Army for three years. Enlisting for three years instead of being drafted for two years guaranteed me a slot in finance. I hoped that this would work out for me since I had added another year on my service commitment to get it.

In 1963 I went to Fort Dix, New Jersey, for basic training. It was tough, but I made it through. I remember when I was into the physical part of basic training I got a severe toothache. The dentist at Fort Dix decided that I needed a wisdom tooth taken out. He proceeded to pull it out using the normal plier type instrument. But it wouldn't come out that way, so he got a chisel and a hammer and proceeded to try and split the tooth. As he directed, I had to put my hand under my jaw, supported by my leg and arm, and hold onto my jaw while he chiseled it otherwise he said he would break my jaw. Just another unbelievable experience.

I can't remember the details, but there was some pressure on us to go through advanced basic training. But I never was into the physical exertion way of life and definitely was not interested in any additional training beyond what was required. As far as I was concerned, it was enough that I had survived the haircut, the KP duty, and the miles of running at double time. Finally, I completed my basic training. What helped me through was visitors day when Ruth and her parents would come for a visit.

Then the assignment orders came out. I was assigned to Fort Benjamin Harrison, Indiana, for finance basic training. I believe this training lasted eight weeks. Ruth came with me. I remember that the training was tougher than I expected. It was a little like a continuation of the regular basic training.

The Army pay at the time was so bad that we could not find a decent place to live. We ended up renting what we called "the red trash can." It was a tiny, red, beat-up trailer. It was in terrible shape and very dirty. The only thing it had going for it was that it was located just outside the entrance road to the installation. Ruth took one look at it and decided to go home. But after the initial shock wore off, she rethought things and decided to persevere. The trailer rent cost more than my total monthly salary, so Ruth had to work also. We had to scrub the trailer from top to bottom to make it livable. We could barely live in it as it was, but we could not afford anything else.

Ruth's mom came for a surprise visit and helped us clean the trailer. One day while Mom Beck was cleaning the windows outside (before we cleaned out the weeds), she stepped into a rusty old pipe and injured her leg. We had to take her to the emergency room for a tetanus shot and to have someone care for her wound. Another unexpected problem was doing laundry. It cost twenty-five cents to wash a load of clothes and ten cents to dry (for ten minutes). When you are making less than a dollar an hour, twenty-five cents is a lot! Money was really tight. We could only afford one dollar monthly for washing clothes, so we used a small canister washing machine that we had to wash our small stuff. This machine was so small that we could use it on top of our kitchen table. It would only wash one set of Army fatigues at a time and it did not wring out the clothes. We had to dry the clothes on a wooden clothes dryer. Ruth had to get a job while we were there. She found one with Lane Bryant in Indianapolis, Indiana. She had to get up at 4 A.M., stand by the highway outside the post, and catch a 5 A.M. bus to the city of Indianapolis. From there she had to walk about two blocks and catch another bus. This bus took her to the final stop. But then she had to walk three blocks to get to work. Her job was to type labels all day. She did all this to be with me.

I had heard that there was a shortage of finance officers in the Army, and since I had my college degree already I could now apply for a direct commission as 2nd Lieutenant Finance Officer. I was only a private, and this was a long shot. Under this plan it was not necessary to go to officer candidate school. However, the Army regulations were that I could not apply for a direct commission until I was physically at my first permanent duty station. Basic training was not a permanent duty station. When I completed my finance basic training, I was assigned to Fort Drum in New York.

KENNETH F. WORTH

I was very happy because this was reasonably close to our home.

But the good news did not last long. I received notice that the orders to assign me to Fort Drum were in error. They were quickly amended, and I found out that I was going to Vietnam. My assignment was to the Special Forces Group at Nha-Trang, Vietnam. It was 1963, and I had heard very little about Vietnam. I didn't have any clear plan for the future, but whatever it might have been, this certainly was not part of it. When my finance training was over, I was sent to my first permanent duty station in Nha-Trang, Vietnam, where I worked in the finance office. Since this was my first permanent duty station, I was now allowed to apply for a direct commission. This was difficult and time consuming to do from Vietnam, but I managed it.

Once again things went amiss. A few months after I applied, I found that my application had been lost somewhere in the Army system. No one could find it. I was advised that I would have to reapply. I considered that, but I did not want to go through the whole process again. So I decided not to submit another application. I was resolved to do my three years as an enlisted man and then get out of the service. I was determined to put the commission out of my mind and not let its loss bother me.

I was stationed in Vietnam in 1963 and 1964 and did the normal year and one day tour. It was an interesting time in many ways. I was there in Vietnam before the big buildup, before the larger amounts of troops were sent to the area. President Kennedy was alive when I arrived in Vietnam, and he was assassinated shortly thereafter. I remember being outside one of the hutches talking to a couple of my buddies when I heard the news about President Kennedy. Ruth remembers being in her dad's car going to the post office to mail me a package when she heard the terrible news on the radio.

While I was in Vietnam I was assigned to the Special Forces Group in Nha-Trang. The president apparently had liked the Special Forces Group, and as a result we had better living conditions than the regular army troops on the other side of the airfield runway which ran the length of the complex. My tour of duty in Vietnam gave me a new appreciation for the Special Forces. If I was in trouble, I would want a Green Beret to rescue me. They are fearless. They have my utmost respect and thanks.

We lived in what was called a "hooch," which was a screened-in building used in place of a tent. There were only 10 people in each hooch. A Vietnamese woman would come daily and make our beds, polish our shoes, and wash our clothes. She used rocks to wash our clothes, so needless to say our uniforms did not last very long. This system caused issues in the country, because though we thought we paid the Vietnamese women only a small amount of money, they were still making far more than their husbands.

We had a mess hall as well in the Special Forces

complex with Vietnamese waiters who would take our order and bring our food to the table. We also had a small movie theater with a snack bar. We saw the latest movies. Our facilities were basic, but they were plush compared with those of the regular troops on the other side of the airfield.

Sometimes we would use the special forces speed boat and go to the Nha-Trang beach. These beaches were beautiful, whitish sand, and it seemed that you could walk out forever in shallow water. We would take our 45-caliber pistols and our AR-15 rifles and shoot at soda cans from the boat. I found that I could pretty well hit the soda cans with shots from the AR-15, but I could not hit a wall with the 45 pistol.

One day we were assigned to guard a high level U. S. government official, who shall remain nameless here, and his daughter who were at Nha-Trang for the day. Our uniform was our bathing suits. I have a picture somewhere of me in my bathing suit standing on the beach by a chopper with my AR-15 rifle guarding the daughter while she was water skiing behind the Special Forces speedboat.

But the conveniences and diversions didn't make our regular job any easier. We still had to go to Saigon on money runs, and we still had to interact with the Special Forces in the field. We would fly into Saigon to pick-up Vietnamese money for our finance office. It must have been a sight—us riding in a big bus to the bank in Saigon with military escorts and coming out with mailbags full

HARD TIMES AND GREAT BLESSINGS

of money. The Vietnamese money was almost as worthless as Monopoly money. The largest Vietnam bill was equivalent to our $5.00 bill. Hence, we needed to use mail bags or something similar to carry enough of it. The bright spot of our trips to Saigon was that our supply sergeant would make sure we flew back from Saigon with ice cream and other goodies for our mess hall and snack bar.

As part of the Special Forces complex security, I had guard duty, which normally involved walking the perimeter fence. Also, I was assigned to a mortar crew. We would practice with live ammunition at times. Fortunately, while I was in Vietnam our complex was not attacked, though we could hear the shooting nearby at times. However, after I left the country I heard that my mortar team blew up the Vietnamese latrine on the complex because of a miscalculation during live ammunition practice. Fortunately, no one was in the latrine at the time.

I am grateful that I did not have to go on many missions while I was in Vietnam. I was assigned to the finance office on the Special Forces complex, and the fighting at that time was mainly in other parts of the country. But I feel for those who saw action every day and have to carry those memories throughout life. When you see a Vietnam veteran, give them a hearty, "Welcome home," and, "Thank you for your service." I do.

There are still questions about the effects of certain chemicals such as agent orange used during the time I was in the country. Was I exposed to any of these environmental agents? Only time will tell.

I remember that I did go on one very interesting and unusual mission. I was selected as a "volunteer" in the strictest Army sense of the term. A general, who shall also remain nameless here, picked a mission force of "volunteers" who were lucky enough to be in our complex at the time. I was one of those picked. It didn't matter to the general if we were Special Forces qualified or not. Apparently, there were a few American soldiers being held hostage in a nearby South Vietnamese military encampment. We were quickly briefed, but we were not given much detail. We only knew that another band of South Vietnamese militants were just outside the encampment waiting to attack it. It was odd, but both the South Vietnamese in the camp and those outside waiting to attack it were both our allies. Because of this, our objective was to go in and rescue the hostages without any fighting if at all possible. What surprised me were the instructions given to us on how to accomplish the mission. First, we had to shave and put on clean uniforms. Then we were to fly to the campsite in helicopters. One chopper would land while the others would circle the camp in a show of force. I would be in a circling chopper. Those in the first chopper would go into the camp and negotiate the release of the hostages. If they were successful, they would set off a green flare and bring the hostages out to the choppers and back to our complex. The mission would then be ended. However, if the negotiations were not successful, a red flare would be set off, and we would spring into action, land, and enter the complex in a "V" formation. In this case, we were to keep our weapons pointed down and not at the captors.

If all this sounds rather a little shaky, hang on. It gets even more bizarre. We were instructed that after we had entered the camp, if we met with resistance from the Vietnamese captors, we were to pick them up gently and set them aside. We were told we could do this because the Vietnamese were small in stature. I'm not making this up. We were further briefed that if a fight did break out, we were to fight our way to a building in the back of the camp where the hostages were being held and take control of the building. Then an Air Force jet would come in and destroy the whole camp with napalm, except for our building. Yeah, right! Then we would come out of the building and board the chopper back to our complex.

Fortunately, the negotiation team was successful, and we saw green smoke. The captors released the hostages and my chopper never had to land there. It was not necessary to implement the rest of the "plan." The mission was over. As we were flying back to our compound, I thought about God's hand of blessing being on my life.

During my stay in Vietnam, I looked forward to the many care packages Ruth sent filled with Slim Jims and other assorted goodies. I would scarf them down quickly. I also gave some of the items to my buddies, especially the Slim Jims. These were so popular that our mess sergeant special ordered them for sale in our snack bar.

Before I went to Vietnam, I bought two tape recorders that were exactly the same. Ruth kept one and I took the other one with me. We made tapes and wrote letters daily to each other. Because of the slow mail system, sometimes we would get a whole pile of letters at one time. Ruth said she usually got a mailbox filled with letters and tapes written over many weeks. I also sent money to a florist near where Ruth lived, and they would deliver flowers to her every month.

The major problem I had in Vietnam was not seeing my wife. I missed her. It seemed that my year there was much longer than the normal year. But the tour did come to an end, and I did come home.

It was a policy of the Army to assign soldiers returning from Vietnam to their choice of installation if possible. This worked out well for me. I requested Fort Monmouth which was close to home. Thankfully, my assignment in finance at Fort Monmouth was approved.

We still needed to supplement my military pay, and Ruth still had to work. She found a job in the parts department at Montgomery Ward. It was a good job for the time, and she worked there until my next assignment and move.

While I was at Fort Monmouth, my grandmother died. She was not feeling well, and then she was frightened by some kids at Halloween. We felt that had an impact on her just before she died. She is with the Lord. Thanks for everything, Grandma.

I wasn't at Fort Monmouth very long when a strange thing happened. I had risen to the grade of Specialist E-5. It was nice to finally get to this level in the enlisted ranks. Normally at that level you do not do KP (kitchen police) duty, but due to a shortage of military personnel I got stuck with this assignment. Just my luck.

Then, first thing in the morning, orders came down from Department of the Army in Washington, D.C. that I was to be discharged that very day and immediately sworn in as a 2nd Lieutenant. No one at Fort Monmouth was expecting this, including me! I had given up on my application for a direct commission when I was in Vietnam and had not mentioned it to anyone at Fort Monmouth. At first no one believed it. Then they didn't understand it. Then they had to get it done. My lost application for a direct commission had not only been found, it had been approved.

Due to scheduling requirements in the Army, I had to be sworn in that day and immediately go on leave. Then I was to report to Fort Benjamin Harrison in Indiana for finance officers training. I did not have to go to officer's candidate school as was normally the case. The Army just gave me the commission. Hard times had come, but this was another of God's great blessings. I thought my application was lost, but God works in strange ways, and it was approved.

The details of my swearing in as an officer still give me a chuckle. The day my unexpected commission arrived, there were no official Army orders in writing and no one could find an officer willing to swear me in without written orders. A warrant officer agreed but was not allowed to do it per Army regulations. Finally, in mid-afternoon a fax came in directing the action be done that day. A colonel agreed to do it, and I was sworn in.

The confusion did not end with the officers. "Specialist Worth" was scheduled to report that morning to Sergeant Jones who was in charge of KP assignments. Since I was in the process of being commissioned, I didn't show for KP. Sergeant Jones was mad, and he called the office I worked in to ask why I had not shown up. He was told that there was no longer a "Specialist Worth," but he could talk to "Lieutenant Worth" if he liked. I must admit I enjoyed that moment. I'm sure I looked funny walking around the installation with the outline of my removed Specialist E-5 patch still showing on my sleeves and the 2nd Lieutenant bars on my collar. As was the tradition, I gave $1.00 to the first enlisted man to salute me.

The direct commission, however, was not fully automatic. I had to decide whether or not to accept it. It required a two year commitment, and I only had nine months left on my tour. I took it. So what had started out as a two year draft commitment turned into four years and three months and five days of military service in the Army. I didn't realize how much being an officer would improve my Army life nor the influence it would have on the rest of my life.

CHAPTER 5
CAREER

It was 1965, and I was stationed at Fort Benjamin Harrison in Indiana as a finance officer. This was a nice assignment after spending a year in Vietnam. This was my first assignment as an officer. I worked in the Allotments and Deposits Operations at the massive Army Finance Center building.

When I first got to Fort Harrison, I went through finance training again. Only this time it was officers training. When my training was over I received my permanent duty assignment and it was a good one. I was assigned to the finance center right there on Fort Harrison. Of course, in my position at the finance center I dealt with only a small portion of the accounting system. But it appeared to me that what this position needed was more of a coordinator or manager rather than an accountant. Nevertheless, I was glad to have such an assignment. The people I worked with were very nice, and the work was very rewarding.

I had another interesting assignment as a Survivors Assistance Officer (SAO) for the family of a soldier who died in an accident during a training exercise. My job as SAO was to assist the family and insure that they received all the benefits they were due by Army regulations. What made this more interesting was that the soldier was a member of an Indian tribe and also an eagle scout in the Boy Scouts. Both groups were there taking turns standing at attention next to the casket honoring the soldier. It was impressive and touching. That was my only SAO duty and it was an honor.

This was the second time the Army had sent me to Fort Benjamin Harrison. The first time I was assigned there I was an enlisted person living in a run-down trailer. This time was different. I was living in the very nice officers quarters on post with all the benefits of being commissioned. I remember that as part of my duties I was to give tours of the impressive finance center with it's "miles of files." Actually, giving these tours ended up being one of the more enjoyable parts of my job. I liked interacting with the people taking the tours. I wonder how the miles of files would go over today in our paperless digital world.

When we moved to Indiana, Ruth had to work again. She took the civil service exam and passed it the first time. Fortunately, she found a secretarial job at the finance center. She worked there until she became pregnant and got sick and physically unable to continue working.

During my off duty time, I ran a Royal Rangers

outpost in the Assembly of God Church in Indianapolis. It was very rewarding to see the boys grow spiritually. We were reaching out to some of the toughest kids around. I didn't realize that I was going into parts of town that I wasn't supposed to go without a military escort.

My oldest daughter Cheryl was born in the military hospital at Fort Benjamin Harrison (so she's a Hoosier!). This was our third pregnancy. Early in our marriage, Ruth had two miscarriages. And this third pregnancy did not end with an easy delivery. Ruth was in labor for 17 hours before Cheryl was born. We were thankful for a beautiful, healthy, baby girl. She was another of God's greatest blessings. The doctor who delivered Cheryl lived in officers quarters near us. When we went to Fort Harrison we still had that 1960 Ford that we bought after our honeymoon. I remember that Lt. Keith Sharkey had the same make and model car. He was living next door in the officers quarters, and we became friends. The Shark, as we called him, mistakenly got in my car one day and tried to start it. It worked! What's more, we then discovered that my keys worked in his car too. I never thought that was possible.

Sharkey was the commander of a company on post. Though we had different assignments, we became friends and got along very well together. One thing we did together was build a small row boat in our back yard. We used the boat a few times and it actually stayed afloat. It was something fun to do. I don't remember what happened to the boat when I left Indiana.

After six years of dependability we traded in our Ford and bought a new 1966 yellow Mustang. It was a beautiful car with spinners on the wheels and a leather interior. It was the nicest car I ever had. I was stopped at a light a few months later when someone in an older car came out of a parking area and smashed into the right side of my car. You can imagine how I felt. To make matters worse, the driver took off. So I took off after her. But she lost me in traffic. When I called the police, they said that since I had left the scene of the accident I was out of luck and could not even get an accident report. I did manage to get her license number and from that found out her address. I reported this to my insurance company who handled it from there. I don't know what the results were on their end, but my insurance company fixed my car.

We enjoyed living in the officers quarters at Fort Harrison. It was like another life being an officer. I had lived on both sides of the street, so to speak, and there was an indescribable difference. Living and working conditions for an officer were so much better than for enlisted personnel.

I was due either to take action to extend my service with a promotion to the rank of captain or get discharged when my tour of duty at Fort Harrison was over. However, I knew that if I stayed in the Army I would be going back to Vietnam. I decided to leave the service. My wife had a difficult

HARD TIMES AND GREAT BLESSINGS

time with the year long separation the first time I had a tour of duty overseas. But the Army had been good to me, and I had no complaints. Having the military experience helped me in my personal life and career for many years to come. Life was good for now.

In 1967, I started working as a civilian at Fort Monmouth, New Jersey. I had sent out numerous applications for positions in different parts of the country, but I really wanted to work at Fort Monmouth or at least in that general area where I grew up. I wanted to stay in the Army as a civilian if I could. Lots of people apply for jobs at Army installations, but I had an advantage in getting a civilian job working for the Army as I was currently an Army officer in a related job.

Then I received a call from the Fort Monmouth personnel office indicating that they wanted to schedule a telephone interview for me with their comptroller for a civilian position with the Army at Fort Monmouth. The interview went very well, and I was selected for a position as auditor.

I did not realize it at the time, but the comptroller had hired me directly without the knowledge or approval of the supervisor in the audit area, Mr. Littleton. What is it that they say about starting off on the wrong foot? It seemed that is what always happened to me. I was selected for this job while I was still in the Army and without an on-site, face-to-face interview. I wore a uniform one day as an Army officer and put on a suit the next day as a civilian.

Perhaps the fact that I just showed up at the office one day without the chief knowing that I was coming or that I was even selected was the reason I did not totally fit in. This was a challenging job with a lot of interesting audits. It was also one of God's blessings to me.

The most interesting audits to me were those of the officers and non-commissioned officers clubs on post. They were an internal control challenge. This was especially true in the area of liquor controls. We had to ensure that liquor was properly handled and controlled from its purchase to its verified destruction.

We bought our first home while I worked at Fort Monmouth. It was a small house in Shark River Hills and cost less than the price of a new car today. It needed some work, but it was not a fixer-upper. We remodeled it inside and out, including painting and tiling the bathroom. It was a very nice first house and was in a nice area. My brother-in-law Bob and his family lived across the street.

We used to hold very large garage sales at our house and the money went to the Royal Rangers group at our church. We were known in the area for driving around and picking up items that were being thrown out. These things would then be sold in our garage sales. These funds covered a portion of the costs for the club's trips and outings.

The audit office where I worked was rather loose from a management perspective. The secretary was even known to cook eggs in the mornings for those auditors who were in the office. But this atmosphere may have been what made the office so effective. In spite of the easy-going environment, most of the auditors' time was spent in the field doing on-site audits. The general rule was that you were not working when you were in the office. It was fine to be in the office writing up an audit report. But most of the auditors got the message and wrote their reports in the field.

One day my supervisor, Mr. Littleton, was driving in his car and leaned over to swat a bug. I'm not sure if he managed to get the bug, but he did manage to launch his car over an embankment and into a parking lot. Fortunately, the lot was empty. Of course, the undercarriage of the car was damaged, and all four tires blew out on impact. But Mr. Littleton was not hurt.

While I was at Fort Monmouth, I had other jobs to make ends meet. I worked for CUTCO selling knives and accessories door-to-door. I discovered that I was a better manager than I was a salesman. I sold a lot of individual pieces and not that many full sets of knives. I had a tendency, for example, to sell two steak knives to a couple instead of a set of six or eight steak knives. I believed in the knives and am still using the ones from my sales kit today. But I was relieved when I was moved from sales to teaching other people how to do presentations to customers.

I also worked for Lerner Shops as an assistant

manager. The store was in a mall, so it had a good volume of people coming in daily. What I actually did there was more of a security guard and closer rather than an assistant manager. I walked the store looking for theft and assisted in closing out the register and locking up.

Another job I had was working at the Garden State Arts Center as a security guard one summer. My brother-in-law Bill already worked there and got me the job. This was very interesting. I walked the perimeter fence near the main building where the shows were performed. My responsibilities included stopping people from coming over the wall. Bill had been working there for years. Unlike me, he often worked backstage, where he met and interacted with the stars. I remember when he took Mom Beck backstage to see Liberace, the famous piano player. She was so excited. This meant so much to her. Liberace was very gracious and signed a picture for her.

I also sold whole-house humidifiers door-to-door with Bill and our mutual friend, Joseph. All the installations were done by Joseph since he was the only one qualified. These humidifiers were nice. They were installed in forced-air furnaces and humidified the whole house. We didn't do this very long because it just wasn't profitable for the time and effort put in.

I had yet another job working with Bill. We delivered appliances for a local appliance store using Bill's truck that he owned for another

HARD TIMES AND GREAT BLESSINGS

business. This work was too hard on my back. Bill started doing all the heavy-end lifting. It was particularly hard delivering refrigerators to upstairs addresses. We both decided to move on to other things.

It was here in New Jersey at the Full Gospel Church that I was first elected to a church board. This was a big responsibility and a real spiritual experience. Over time, I would serve on church boards in Pennsylvania, New Jersey and Massachusetts.

While I was still working at Fort Monmouth, an agreement was made between Fort Monmouth and Fairleigh Dickinson University (FDU) to run special MBA (master's in business administration) degree classes at Fort Monmouth. I was one of the first to apply for admission. Growing up I had never placed much importance on my education. Even in college, my attitude had not changed much. As a result, my Grade Point Average (GPA) from high school and from college was not very good. However, I knew that both FDU and Fort Monmouth wanted their cooperative program and the new MBA program to work, and I saw this as a good opportunity to advance my career. I believe the big push to get the program off the ground resulted in lenient admission procedures. I was accepted!

It was tough working full time while going for my master's degree, but I did it. One thing that helped me a lot was that most of the classes were held at Fort Monmouth. I only had a few classes where I had to drive to FDU, which was a three-hour round trip. In 1976 I graduated from FDU with an MBA in management. This was quite an accomplishment for me considering my historic lack of interest in education in general. This was another of God's blessings to me and a definite help to my future career.

About this time, we had a dangerous encounter on the road. It was the end of the work day as Ruth, Cheryl, and I neared the Fort. I had taken a day's leave, but I had to go into the office to pick up an important audit report for review for an exit conference the next day. Ruth had just taken Cheryl out of her car seat (she was fussing) and placed her on her lap. It wasn't much of a lap as we were expecting our second child in about a month.

Cars were bumper-to-bumper going the other way out of the Fort, but very few were going in as I was. Suddenly, a driver coming out of the Fort decided to risk a fast left turn into a street just in front of my car. Here he came, driving on the wrong side of the street right at us trying to slip in the side road before we got there. He miscalculated. I jammed on the brakes and got stopped, but I did not have time to back up. His car hit us head on with most of the impact on the passenger's side. The impact drove Ruth and Cheryl into the padded dash of the car. It was a miracle that they were not seriously hurt. However, Cheryl's nose made a permanent indentation in the dash. Both Ruth and Cheryl were taken to the hospital to be checked out for any possible internal injuries. They checked out fine. The car was almost totaled. I had the car fixed and then traded it in.

My younger daughter, Julia, was born in 1968 in Neptune, New Jersey. Ruth and I had been blessed with Cheryl and now were blessed again with Julia. As I am writing this, they are grown women. Both are college graduates and married. Cheryl and her husband Howard have three sons. Julia and her husband Rob are both in the ministry. Rob is currently completing his PhD in Renewal Studies. We are so proud of them and all they have accomplished.

As our family grew, our two bedroom home in Shark River Hills was getting too small. We needed more room. We bought a really nice large corner lot in Wall Township, New Jersey. At the time, it looked like we would stay at Fort Monmouth and retire there some day. Since we were planning on staying there permanently, Fred Beck, my multi-talented father-in-law, drew for us plans for a large ranch house. I was my own general contractor. Actually, it could be said that I was a puppet general contractor and Fred was the puppeteer. He knew what to do and when to do it. He was exceptional in all areas needed to build a house from the ground up. I wish Fred had written his life story. He had lived through the Great Depression and had studied in the school of hard knocks. He had built at least three houses himself. Fred and I did the work that we could and contracted out the rest.

KENNETH F. WORTH

I remember one day a man named Hipolet came walking around the corner looking for work. We ended up hiring him on the spot to install the cedar shingles on the whole house. He did the job for $500.00 labor and did an excellent job. The contractor who did the framing charged $1.00 per square foot for labor. We did the whole house this way and saved money.

A contractor who specialized in insulation did the whole house for less than we could have bought the material. He bought the insulation by the train load and therefore could do the job more economically. When our house was completed, it exceeded even our expectations. But we didn't know we would not be staying there.

Over time, I had become friends with Grant Stockton, another auditor. Grant was not one of the "in group" around our place of work, but I didn't care. Grant was my friend and would remain so. I did my job and was given great performance reviews but did not advance as quickly as I could have. I realized, over time, that I would have to leave the Fort Monmouth area if I was to get a promotion. To stay would be a detriment to my career.

I applied for positions at other installations. One of those applications was to New Cumberland Army Depot (NCAD) in Pennsylvania in an organization called the U. S. Army Security Assistance Center (USASAC). This job involved foreign military sales. I was interviewed and offered a position as senior auditor. I was excited at the prospect of this interesting job and getting back in the career advancement channels. I accepted the job, and we moved to Pennsylvania.

CHAPTER 6
THE ARSENAL

When I was selected for the position of senior auditor in Pennsylvania, we had all the problems related to moving from one state to another state. We knew the drill from prior moves, but it never got easier. If anything, it kept getting harder.

When the time came to actually move to Pennsylvania, I moved first and brought the family later. I found a room in a boarding house in Hershey, PA. Hershey was a neat town with its chocolate factory and Hershey kisses-shaped street lights. I took the factory tour many times and went to Hershey Park, but it was no fun without my family. I only stayed there a short while, and then I moved to an apartment in Enola, PA.

The Army paid for our move, but as our multi-stage move dragged on, the money we had received kept decreasing. That encouraged me to keep looking for more economical places to live. Ruth and the kids came to live with me in Enola. Ruth still had to work in order for us to make ends meet.

KENNETH F. WORTH

She found a job in the Fuels Division of the General Material and Petroleum Activity (GMPA) area on New Cumberland Army Depot (NCAD).

While we were living in Enola, we had some interesting experiences. One Saturday we had to get out of the apartment quickly because one of the kids in an apartment two doors down set fire to his place. Fortunately, no one was hurt and the fire was put out quickly, limiting damage to the one apartment. Another day we woke up to find that the sewer had backed up into our bathtub. This was a mess that happened a few times during our stay there. Another problem living there was that our kids were being picked on in school and at the complex pool. We did not know the magnitude of the problem until years later. We learned that Cheryl had watched out after her younger sister like a bulldog.

While we were in Enola, we bought a house in Boiling Springs, PA. Financially, things really got tough for a while. We were carrying our old house in New Jersey, our new house in Pennsylvania, and an apartment in Pennsylvania all at the same time. We have never sold a house quickly, and this was not an exception. It took us about eight months to sell our house in New Jersey. Then we left Enola and moved to our new house in Boiling Springs and stayed there until we finally left Pennsylvania.

This was an interesting place to live. It was in a development that was two miles up a heavily wooded mountain road. This was a potential problem. In the event of a forest fire, this road was the

HARD TIMES AND GREAT BLESSINGS

only way in or out of the mountain. This was also a very real problem in heavy rain or snow. It was a beautiful place to live, but when it rained hard the road at the bottom of the mountain flooded and it was dangerous or impossible to get through.

They say not to drive through water flooded across the road, but I, like so many others, did not listen. I once went through some water that was rushing across the road. It was deeper than it looked. I lost track of where I was on the road. Trying to find the center of the road, I opened the car door to look at where the water level was. That was a mistake. The water was much higher than I thought. Water poured into the car through the open door. I quickly shut the door, but now I was concerned that the car engine would die from water submerging the exhaust pipe. Somehow I made it through and drove up the mountain. When I braked to turn into my street, the water came rushing up from the back seat area and wet my feet and everything in the front. This was a mess to clean up and dry.

When it snowed we would carefully drive down the mountain because it was easy to slide. If we had to go up the mountain, we would try to hit the steeply inclined road with some speed. We usually could not make it all the way up so we would leave the car where it stopped and start walking. Many people living on the mountain had four wheel drive cars and would pick us up and take us home. Often when it snowed, the street in front of our house would be closed so the kids could sled down it.

One day I noticed a vintage car in my neighbor's driveway. It had a familiar look to it. He was going to restore it. I went over to see it and discovered that it was a 1948 Ford. Further examination showed that it was the same model and year as my first car. Talk about feeling old. My first car was now an antique.

While I was a senior auditor at USASAC an interesting thing happened. We were doing a very large audit of some specific foreign military sales contracts and our chief, Drew Templeton, was on vacation at Disney World in Florida. It was determined that he needed to be back at the office to deal with a specific problem that he had been personally handling. Headquarters made the arrangements and Drew was paged at Disney World and immediately flown back to USASAC. Drew now had a story to tell about the day he was pulled out of Disney World and flown back to work.

At work things were going well. We did audits of literally billions of dollars in foreign military sales. I was Acting Chief of the Internal Review and Audit Compliance (IRAC) office for a short time while the chief was at long-term training. This was a very good experience which helped me in career development and in getting my next position in USASAC.

The position of Budget Office Chief came open, and I applied for it. The budget office was performing very well and had well-qualified people, but their relationship with top management was somewhat strained. I got the job. This was an excellent opportunity giving me a budget background which I did not previously have.

I was able to repair the strained relationship between the budget office and top management. It was here that I began to show my managerial skills and the fact that they actually worked. It was a significant boost in my career advancement and potential.

At work, a situation developed whereby the Deputy Comptroller saw the Chiefs of Offices under him getting together occasionally in their offices. He believed they were talking about him behind his back. I was one of those chiefs. However, we were not talking about him. We just got along very well together and got together for coffee.

One morning when I arrived at work I noticed that the door to my office was missing. Soon it was apparent to everyone that the doors to all the Chiefs' offices were off. They had been removed overnight. It appears that the deputy thought that taking the doors off would stop the Chiefs from meeting together. He had a very unusual management style and way of dealing with this problem.

As time went on, I found that from a career perspective, it was time to look for new opportunities. I had come to USASAC as a senior auditor and had been promoted to Budget Office Chief. This was another of God's blessings. But I could see that I had advanced as far as I could go at USASAC without going to headquarters near Washington, D. C.

I applied to other installations, including the Pentagon. Though I didn't want to go to the Washington, D. C., area, I applied for the job at the Pentagon because I knew that this is where the highest level jobs were. I was only partially qualified for the position, but I made the cut to be in the final three candidates, and I went to the Pentagon for a personal interview. The interview went well, but I did not get the job. However, the selecting official did apparently make the right choice. I had foreign military sales background in the Army, but the person who was selected had a similar background dealing with all three branches of military service.

After that interview, I did hear from the Pentagon about other jobs but I did not apply. That was the country boy in me coming out again. The truth was that I wanted to avoid the urban world of Washington, D. C.

I have been through quite a few interviews and have done very well in all of them. I did not get some of the positions because I had a tendency to shoot high and apply for jobs for which I did not have sufficient experience (at least on paper). I usually ended up among the top three candidates.

Then I found that I was being considered for a position in Watertown, Massachusetts. The job interview for the position of Director, Resource

HARD TIMES AND GREAT BLESSINGS

Management (DRM) at the Watertown Arsenal in Watertown was a very unusual experience. (The facility went by various names over the years. I will just call it "the Arsenal.") It became obvious to me that top management at the Arsenal was putting heavy emphasis on getting this selection right.

I had never been to that area, but I really wanted the job and was prepared to jump through hoops to get it. Looking back, I realize that I rather enjoyed the unique interview process. I was very interested in the inner workings of interviews in general. In fact, I would later teach a course at the Arsenal called "How To Be Successfully Interviewed." However, I could not foresee the unusual interview techniques that I discovered for the DRM position.

It all started when I first applied for the DRM position. My application got me the interview. In the Army, to apply for a position you fill out a form as opposed to submitting a resume. So you need to be innovative to stand out among the other applicants. I had a reputation for preparing Army job applications that were effective and resulted in job interviews. My application survived the screening process, and I was selected for a personal interview. I don't know how many others were considered for the position but I believe many were involved in the process.

The interview process began when I received a telephone call requesting an interview with the installation commander, Colonel Johnson. I have been through quite a few interviews and feel that I know the process and techniques fairly well. But this was an unusual interview. The Colonel's interview lasted well over two hours and covered all aspects of the position requirements and my background. The commander was interested in my managerial approach under various scenarios. The interview went very well. I felt that my answers to all the questions were accurate and well received and I handled the interview extremely well. I had to make sure that my qualifications and management abilities were discussed. It felt like I was in charge of the interview.

Then the next day I had another telephone interview with the civilian deputy director, Dr. Sneider. That interview also lasted well over two hours and covered much of the same areas. There was emphasis in the interview on my view and methods in providing support services. Dr. Sneider seemed to be more skilled in the interview process, but I still felt that I had overall control of the interview. In both interviews it became clear to me that this position was going to be filled from outside the organization.

The in-house perception of services provided by the DRM was not good. I had the impression that the actual work was excellent but the timeliness of responses to questions and the personal interface with top management needed to be improved. The new DRM would have to shoulder the burden of an organization perceived as under-performing. What is important here is the word perceived. In reality

HARD TIMES AND GREAT BLESSINGS

the DRM staff was doing excellent work—much better than the top managers realized. All that was necessary was to interact more quickly with the top managers and the perception of service received would increase favorably. This was my kind of job. The DRM would also be responsible for changing from one accounting system to another. This would include moving the staff, that was familiar with the old system, over to the new one that was being implemented.

The facility military commander was responsible for the operational portion of the Arsenal where the DRM position was located. The civilian Director was responsible for the laboratories and research and development programs. I would have to work very closely with both of them.

The day after the second interview, I received a call from the Arsenal personnel office. They wanted to schedule an interview at the Arsenal within the week. I was flown in to Watertown for a series of interviews at the Arsenal. When I arrived I was brought to an inner office and different people came in to interview me. As I recall, there were about ten people who interviewed me that day. One laboratory director came and interviewed me in a traditional interview style. Then another director came. Then another interviewer came who sat down, looked me in the eye, and said, "I don't want to be here, but they told me I had to interview you." Then another and so on. The equal employment officer came. The commander came and took another quick shot as did the civilian deputy director. Then I was taken into a large, plush office to meet the civilian director. This was the person who really ran the installation.

It was a tiresome but rewarding day. The marathon interviews were over. I felt good about the day and enjoyed the interview process because I felt I had been able to adapt to each interviewer. I waited. Finally, I was selected for the position as Director, Resource Management. I got along well with all the commanders and laboratory directors during my whole career at the Arsenal.

Our move to Massachusetts was quite an experience. I went ahead but Ruth stayed behind and joined me a few weeks later after I found an apartment in Natick, Massachusetts. I needed another car to use in Massachusetts while Ruth kept our current car in Pennsylvania. So, I called a new car dealer and made my deal including buying the car over the phone. I told the sales manager that I needed a car and didn't have time to shop. I gave him my social security number and he got the car loan approved. Two days later I picked up the car and saw it for the first time. It was ready to drive away. It was a 1983 Chevy Cavalier and the only car I ever bought over the phone.

I did not realize when I took the job that I was putting myself in what could have been a sticky situation. Bill Taylor was acting in the DRM job and was extremely well liked by the staff. Many of the personnel had assumed that he would get the

HARD TIMES AND GREAT BLESSINGS

DRM job. The staff was not happy that someone from outside was coming in to take the job. What made matters worse was that Bill was in the hospital at the time. He was still there when he was told he did not get the job. I did not know about any of this at the time, but it made my job harder, at least at first. However, I was a manager, and I saw this job as an opportunity to shine and significantly improve operation of the Resource Management areas of responsibility.

As the DRM, I had operational control of critical areas of the arsenal. My staff had a service reputation that needed a significant improvement in a short time frame. Top management perceived two problems. First, that overall service was not up to par. Second, there was the expectation that the change to a new accounting system would not happen on time or properly. This was even more important because of the intense interest shown by headquarters in meeting the dates established for completion of the accounting change.

My management style was a perfect fit for this situation. I just needed to get by the fact that Bill Taylor did not get the position. That worked itself out over time, and I was accepted into the DRM position by most of the people we serviced and those who worked with me.

I used the MBWA management philosophy (Manage By Walking Around), making sure that I talked about only positive things on my "walk abouts" and did not talk about problems. I practiced what I preached and tackled the perceived problems first not necessarily the most important operationally. Perception is reality.

It became apparent very quickly that an infusion of new personnel in key positions was necessary to provide the staff some overall guidance and support. I brought in a new budget officer with substantial experience in the new accounting system.

I brought in a management analyst from outside the organization to do a management study and recommend changes. I also had my own ideas for change, but I realized that the changes had to come from the staff members themselves in order to be effective and receive their support.

The management analyst did her job and came up with a report of recommendations for procedural and organizational change. This worked very well because one of my management philosophies was to find ways to get my staff to recommend to me exactly what I wanted to do anyway. I could then implement ideas which appeared to be coming from the staff and which the staff would support as their own.

It worked perfectly this time. I met with my staff and let them know I was implementing the changes they recommended. I got tremendous support and cooperation from the staff, proving once again that perception is the rule. What you think is real is real to you.

Over the next few months our service reputation soared. I really enjoyed working as the DRM at the

HARD TIMES AND GREAT BLESSINGS

Arsenal. It had been a good career move. Meanwhile, Ruth continued to work. She applied for and got a position in the Arsenal's contracts office. As time went on, she got a promotion working for one of the laboratory directors. She worked there under several laboratory directors until she retired in 1995.

Then another position opened up at the Arsenal that provided another promotion for me. It was another area with perceived service deficiencies and another position for which I did not have the technical qualifications. Taking on this type of challenge was what I loved and was good at. I believe that I do best in a problem situation where there is no way to go but up. I applied for and got the position of Chief, Management Information Systems Office (MISO) at the Arsenal. This gave me operational control over computer operations. I did not have a background in the computer area, but I got the job because of my proven managerial accomplishments at the Arsenal.

MISO needed an overhaul. The service reputation within the commander and director areas needed improvement. Actually, the major problem was a perceived lack of timely service to top management based on MISO just not getting to the problem quickly enough. Once we got there we fixed the problems quickly and accurately. This problem was handled quickly with a change in policy. I remember briefing my staff and informing them of my operational philosophy regarding service. I explained that everyone at the Arsenal was to be treated equally, but the front office was to be treated a little more equally than the others. The MISO service reputation improved significantly in a short period of time. Once again I had a staff that was very skilled and just needed some guidance.

That reminds me of the "tanker," Major Legune. He had been recently reassigned from the tank command to one of the laboratories at the Arsenal. One day, he got some work he wasn't happy with from the systems area of MISO. It was a minor problem which was easily corrected. The major chewed out Mary, one of my staff, who had done the work. I heard about it and decided to take action.

Those aware of the situation were puzzled at my approach. I invited the major to lunch. At lunch we had a chance to discuss the situation in some detail. We had a man-to-man discussion during which I explained to the major that he was no longer a tanker dealing with military personnel. I informed him that he could not treat civilians that way, especially my people. We came to an understanding. The major apologized to Mary and thereafter he got along very well with her and with the rest of my staff. Moreover, my staff appreciated my support for Mary. It was a win-win-win situation.

Then, another new position was developed at the Arsenal which included all information systems. This covered essentially everything on the installation except the research laboratories. I applied for

HARD TIMES AND GREAT BLESSINGS

and got the dual position as Director of Information Management (DOIM) and Commander, USA Information Systems Command (USAISC). The same service reputation perception was true for this position. It needed to be improved in many areas. This was right up my alley.

Over the next few months, I made organizational and operational changes to improve service. The reputation of the DOIM organization was continually getting better. This tied into another management philosophy of mine which was to take jobs managing areas where there are perceived problems. I feel you can make improvements quickly in those situations. You can't help but look good especially if you tackle and resolve the perceived problems first.

One problem I ran into though was that I was responsible to provide service to the commander and director as the DOIM, but I was not under their operational control as the commander of USAISC at Watertown. In other words, the commander or director could task me to complete a project but they could not direct me how to do it. This situation, combined with my independent attitude and the confidence I had in my management abilities, soon produced conflicts between me and the top management on the Arsenal. They were used to having things done their way and I was just given the authority to do them my way. I knowingly burned all my bridges behind me. However, service continued to improve.

KENNETH F. WORTH

One example was in the technical reports area. Laboratory directors would submit technical reports and we would review them prior to publication. When I came into the job, we were behind about one year in processing these reports. One of my first management actions was to move one authorized position from the technical reports area to my office.

The director of the laboratories heard about the action I had taken and was upset. After discussing the issue, we were unable to come to an agreement. However, I moved the position as I planned. Within a few months, the technical reports backlog was gone and that section was looking for work. I had changed processing procedures and contracted out most of the review workload. Another problem solved.

While I was the commander of USAISC at Watertown, another position opened up back in Fort Monmouth, New Jersey. Even though it was essentially the same position as I currently had at the Arsenal, it would be a promotion for me due to the size and complexity of the job. It was a higher government job grade. I applied for the position and once again made it to the final three. I was looking forward to the interview process.

Ruth and I decided to take a trip to the area as it had been quite a while since I was there and since it was less than a three hour trip to get there. We were taken aback by the changes in the area since we had last been there. Cars were everywhere. To this country boy, the changes were not for the better. The cost of living had also skyrocketed. We went back home and I called Fort Monmouth and took my name off the list of candidates for the position. We will never know what the outcome would have been, but I'm glad I stayed a country boy.

My focus on my career was interrupted one day when I got a surprise call from my brother Carl. I had lost touch with him for a while, but I knew he was in the South somewhere. In years past, I was used to getting calls from Carl when he was in trouble. He had really messed up his life. I and my family had continued to pray for Carl all through the years. However, when he talked to me on this day, he said something that I admit that I was not expecting. He dropped a bomb on me. He had accepted Jesus as his personal savior!

It seemed unreal, impossible. At first, I didn't believe him. We pray, and when the answer comes, we question it. Where is our faith? Then it hit me that he was actually telling the truth. Our prayers were answered. Hallelujah! Anyone who knew Carl and how he had acted over the years would say it was a real miracle.

From then on Carl changed. He served God and put the rest of us to shame. We watched him grow in the Lord. He began to sing gospel songs in his church, and then he began to sing wherever he could. He loved the southern "sing-ins." He served God with all his being. You couldn't be anywhere with Carl for any time without him talking about the

KENNETH F. WORTH

Lord. Carl died on July 3, 2001. He is with Jesus.

Through much of the time that I worked at the Watertown Arsenal, the facility was on the military base closure list and was fighting for its existence. Everything was done that could be done to keep the Arsenal open but, finally, the decision to close it became permanent. The fight was over. A long, impressive history of accomplishments would be left behind to history and to the memories of those who had worked there over the years.

Once the decision to close was official, another new civilian position that would function in cooperation with the base's military commander was established to exercise operational control of the entire installation through closure. I applied for the position. Remember that I burned my bridges behind me. Based on that, I probably should not have applied for the position. But, as was my custom, I applied for a job that appeared to be over my head and that I never could get politically.

Well, God really does have a sense of humor. Miraculously, I got the job as Site Operations Director (SOD) and ended up with operational control of the entire installation. I had burnt my bridges, but God put them back up. This was another of His blessings to me. I was honestly surprised when I got selected for the position.

When I asked why I was selected instead of someone with more technical environmental and closure experience, I was told it was because I would not overreact and not shoot the messenger

HARD TIMES AND GREAT BLESSINGS

when problems with closure came. The problems did come, and we did resolve them.

Since the Arsenal had a research and development mission, the cleanup for closure was a herculean task. The staff eventually decreased from over five hundred to a streamlined closure staff of twenty-six. We closed the Arsenal in a very efficient and professional way that was considered to be an example of how to close an installation.

A lot of interesting and unusual things happened at the Arsenal almost on a daily basis. One day one of the laboratories had a lunchtime barbecue. However, that particular day was overcast, and soon after the barbecue started it began to rain. Key lab personnel made a decision to solve the problem by taking the grill, still burning, into the laboratory building and up the elevator into an open space area. As you can imagine, it turned out that this was not a good decision. The burning grill cooked the food, but it also set off the fire alarms in the building. The result was that the building had to be evacuated and fire trucks came screaming onto the Installation with sirens blasting to put out the "fire." Needless to say, the laboratories did not barbecue indoors after that.

One event that happened before I was SOD illustrates the kind of strange things that sometimes happened at the Arsenal. Flocks of pigeons had decided to make the gigantic supply building their home. From here, they ran pooh-bombing raids on the supply areas and personnel below. It seems that everything was tried to get rid of the pigeons and their droppings, all to no avail. Nothing worked. Then, over one weekend most of the pigeons suddenly disappeared. Coincidently, there were numerous windows broken out around the upper regions of the building. Someone who worked at the Arsenal had apparently come in over the weekend with a shotgun and blasted both the pigeons and the upper windows where they nested. The windows were replaced and the pigeon problem went away. But like the barbecue fiasco, the tale of the pigeon massacre became part of Arsenal lore.

During the closure of the Arsenal, there were many interesting sights to see. This was especially true of the environmental cleanup actions which were necessary. I remember the men dressed in their full-body protective garments and masks. What a sight! I wondered what the people of Watertown thought was going on inside the Arsenal fences. It looked much more ominous than it was. The contractors had to dress for the worst scenarios even if the conditions did not necessitate it.

I also remember the "march of the trucks." Hundreds of trucks came on the installation as part of the environmental remediation project to pick up loads of dirt and transport it off the Arsenal. Then the trucks came back with loads of new, clean dirt to replace what they had taken out. It was some sight to see the steady stream of the biggest dump trucks I have ever seen lumbering in and out of the facility.

The commander's house on post is a southern

HARD TIMES AND GREAT BLESSINGS

mansion-type building which is on the National List Of Historical Places. Commanders still lived in it until shortly before the base closed for good. When VIPs came they were given the grand tour of the house. Command level parties were held there. It was impressive and one of the better officers quarters in the Army. But the house had its quirks. Rumor was that there was a ghost living in the attic. Supposedly, if you were outside the house looking at the top window you might get to see him. Apparently, my schedule did not coincide with the ghost's, and I never saw him at the window.

When I became the SOD, I knew we had a massive task ahead of us. We not only had to oversee the everyday operations of a military installation with over 500 personnel, but we also had to coordinate closing the installation and bringing the staff down to a final closure staff of twenty-six. We even had a small nuclear reactor that had to be disassembled and removed. Not a piece of cake.

No one knew it at the time, but I came close to not accepting the SOD position. I felt confident in my managerial abilities, but I knew I didn't have the technical environmental background needed to complete the mission. Fortunately, and this was the deciding factor in my decision, we had assembled an excellent base closure staff. I don't believe there could have been any better. Everyone put in the extra effort needed even though by doing so they were doing away with their own jobs. This was a negative incentive environment, yet they did the job with class. Thanks to all of you who made my life at the Arsenal a tremendous success. I appreciate it!

I always said that I would not be the last person out the door stopping to lock up. I chose to retire before that day came. I took some leave time, and then, on November 1, 1997, after thirty-five years working for the Department of the Army (most of it as a civilian), my retirement became official. The installation was officially closed about nine months later and turned over to its new owner. Another chapter of my life had closed. The next was about to begin.

CHAPTER 7
RETIRED

Before I retired, Ruth and I had decided that we wanted to move to the Amish farmland area in Lancaster County, PA. We had been there on many visits over the years. These visits had been especially frequent when we lived in Boiling Springs, which is close to Lancaster county. So, more than two years before my retirement date, we started looking for land in "Amish country." It was difficult finding a piece of land that met our requirements. We wanted lots of trees, level ground, and a spot right among the Amish farms. Not many such lots exist. Most of those that do are owned by the Amish, and they are often sold to other Amish within the community. The "English," which is what the Amish call everyone who is not Amish, often don't have an opportunity to buy this land. However, we worked with an excellent real estate agent.

I remember the trip we took from Massachusetts to Pennsylvania to close the deal on our lot. Normally the trip took about eight hours, but this time we encountered severe fog most of the way. It got so bad we could not see the road. We had to crawl along. Looking back, we should have turned around and rescheduled the closing, but we kept on going. It took us about fifteen hours to get there, almost doubling the normal time. We did close on our lot, and that made the trip worthwhile.

I designed our house on my computer and put the plans and specifications out for bid. It was a custom ranch house all on one floor with wide doorways and halls and no stairs except to the cellar. We were thinking ahead and made it extremely handicapped-friendly even though we were not handicapped at the time. Little did we know how good a decision that was.

I could not believe it—there was a $50,000 difference between the three bids that came back on building the house. We looked at each bid and selected our builder. He was the lowest bidder, but that was not the only criterion which we used in making our selection. I believe he was the lowest bidder because he and his sons did a lot of the hands-on work and needed less sub-contractors than the other bidders. Our decision was made. We awarded the contract and got down to building the house.

Meanwhile, another problem was coming—since we were selling our home in Millis, Massachusetts we were required to have the septic tank inspected. Our septic system failed the test. This was a real surprise as it had apparently been

HARD TIMES AND GREAT BLESSINGS

working fine. Seventeen thousand dollars and a new leeching field later, it passed. This was a financial disaster. After all the problems with the septic system we had to lower the price of the house in order to sell it.

It was quite a task to coordinate the building of a house in Pennsylvania from another state eight hours away. We had to drive back and forth across a lot of empty countryside and wanted to make sure we had a dependable car, so we bought a 2001 Ford Taurus and traded in our 1995 Taurus with 120,000 miles on it. We moved out of the Millis house in mid October, 1997, and stayed temporarily in a motel in Lancaster, PA. It was really a tight squeeze getting the new house ready in time. Early in the morning on the very day we had decided to move in, the builder had told me that he needed another few days to get everything done. "No problem," I told him, "we are going to stay at your house until you get done!" The builder suddenly discovered his ability to work miracles, and the house was completed by evening when we moved in. Talk about close! The inspector was issuing the occupancy permit as we finished moving in. In spite of all the hassle that went along with building the new house, we were glad that we did it. I had it built according to my specifications, and the contractors did a great job. We are still happy here, and we will leave only if we are carried out or can't physically take care of ourselves. We thank God daily for our home which is another of His great blessings.

KENNETH F. WORTH

We moved into our house in Lancaster County on November 2, 1997, the day after I officially retired. After we got settled in, it did not take long before I started getting restless. After my high energy days managing and closing the Arsenal, I became bored. I needed something to do to feel useful. My daughter Julia and I started talking about launching an Internet business selling Amish quilts and crafts. After all, I was in the middle of Amish country in Lancaster County. After some research, Julia and I decided to go ahead with our plan. In November, 1999, we started Worth Crafting at worthcrafting.com.

It took a few months to get recognized by the Internet search engines and to get all the administrative work done that was involved in starting a business. That and other administrative responsibilities were under Julia's care. She also did all the actual programming and systems maintenance on the web site. My responsibility was to coordinate with the Amish suppliers to get them to sell us quality products wholesale and to coordinate the shipping and order-filling processes. In short, I became the interface with the Amish.

It took a substantial amount of time to coordinate with the Amish suppliers. The Amish community was just being introduced to the Internet market, and most of them were not familiar with how the Internet worked. Since the Amish don't have phones and computers in their homes, I had to contact them in person by driving to their houses or stores. With a few exceptions, when we sold something online I had to drive an average of fifteen minutes to drop off the order with an Amish craftsman or store. We learned to live with this as an operational procedure and expense.

We worked on a handshake basis with the Amish suppliers. There were no signed contracts, just our word. We enjoyed working with the Amish and soon we had many products. Eventually, we would have over one hundred items on our web site.

We used an innovative business plan that allowed us to maintain no inventory. We received payment up front at the point of sale. We took the computer generated order form to the Amish craftsman who filled the order and shipped the items out. The Amish would bill us the wholesale price plus shipping and handling fees as agreed upon. They billed us when they wanted to, and we would pay them immediately upon receipt of their bill. We had an excellent reputation for fast payment. We dealt with many Amish suppliers and got along well with all of them.

I enjoyed knowing and working with the Amish. The Amish wholesale craft shows were very nice as they would display literally hundreds of craft items made in the area. Also, the auctions held in the area were impressive. The highlight of most auctions was the quilt sale. You could get a good price on a quality Amish quilt and many other Amish-made items. We became good friends with a few of the Amish, especially with our primary quilt shop supplier in Ronks, Pennsylvania.

Our business did well, but over time it did not bring in sufficient profits to justify the amount of work involved. Moreover, both Julia and I were not well. In March, 2006, we shut down Worth Crafting. It had been fun, but it was over. There were new challenges to deal with.

CHAPTER 8
TRIALS AND BLESSINGS

My older brother, Carl, had died July 3, 2001, at age sixty-five. Prior to this, I had some minor shaking, primarily in my legs. This concerned me, but I had tried to convince myself that it was nothing. However, at my brother Carl's funeral, my family noticed a significant increase in my shaking. My most notable symptoms were tremors, mainly in the left side of my body, my hands, and my legs. My left arm would hang and not swing when I walked. Ultimately, the symptoms would get worse and the tremors would spread to both sides. When it began, I knew something was wrong but I didn't know what it was. But I realized that I couldn't ignore it any longer.

My initial visit to my family doctor did not identify exactly what was wrong. He sent me to a neurologist for a more thorough diagnosis. On my first visit, the neurologist did comprehensive tests, including a substantial symptoms interview. He diagnosed me as having Parkinson's Disease (PD).

KENNETH F. WORTH

It hit me hard. Very hard. I was only sixty-two. I felt sorry for myself and asked the "Why me?" question many times. Then I began to look around and see many others with PD worse off than me and without the many blessings God had bestowed on me. Now I see a blessing in my adversity and God's controlling hand throughout.

Dealing with PD became a journey with its own unique set of challenges. I learned that the Parkinson's diagnosis is a judgment call on the part of the doctor, since there is no one blood test or other diagnostic test that allows a final accurate determination. This is a progressive disease that affects different people with different symptoms and at different rates of progression. You can live a fairly long time with Parkinson's, but your quality of life will continue to decrease until you die. Parkinson's has no mercy and is no respecter of persons. There are five stages to the disease. In my case, subsequent visits to the doctor would result in a determination that I was in stage four of five. Not encouraging information to hear.

On one occasion, when I went to my neurologist for a routine visit, I was informed of two things. First, my neurologist was relocating to Florida where he could do better financially. That meant that I would have to switch to another doctor within the same practice. Second, the practice would no longer take my insurance. That would mean that I had to find an altogether different practice. Hard times. There was a very real shortage of neurol-

HARD TIMES AND GREAT BLESSINGS

ogists in our area to go to for Parkinson's. I was told I would have to go at least an hour away to find another doctor, and even then wait a long time for an appointment.

In the midst of this situation, and just at the right time, came a blessing. I turned sixty-five and went on Medicare. Because of that, I could stay with the same medical practice and keep full coverage, and I found another neurologist in the office who could treat me. It is interesting how God's plan works. Life seemed cruel and unjust, but God was (and is) with me. I don't think I could go through the PD process without Him.

There is nothing "fortunate" about Parkinson's, but I do count myself fortunate in that I only got PD later in life. I feel for everyone with this debilitating disease but especially for those who get it at an early age. I can't believe that I am in stage four of five Parkinson's stages. I don't feel that I am that far along. It seems like it would be more accurate to say that I am in stage three. I've talked to others who have Parkinson's and found that most did not even know that there were stages in the disease.

The hardest part of this journey is knowing that PD will not get better but will continue to progress. Through all this, I realize that I have to live day by day. When I feel sorry for myself, I am reminded of those worse off than me and look at my many blessings.

God has given me great family support. Ruth is the best wife God ever created. She takes care of me and I take care of her. She has physical problems that make it difficult for her to get around herself let alone take care of me. But she still manages. I have two married daughters. Cheryl lives in Texas and would relocate to take care of me in a second should the need arise. Julia and her husband Robby, moved in with us over a year ago and are taking excellent care of us. They lived three hours away in Williamsburg, Pennsylvania, where they pastored a church. They had to leave everything to come and live with us. This is a great blessing from God. I know that whatever life brings, He will always take care of me.

Ruth's history of physical problems has also been a great challenge for us. Among other things, she has had major kidney and knee operations. However, her most recent medical problems have included a growth on the brain and two bouts with different cancers. These are our major concerns regarding her health because they leave her more susceptible to a recurrence. She will have to be checked often.

You've heard the saying, "When it rains, it pours." That has seemed to be the case with my health over the last few years. In May of 2007, I went to my family doctor with chest discomfort. I had no real pain, just discomfort. I thought it was acid reflux, which I had before. To my surprise, it was my heart. The doctor immediately sent me to a heart specialist who quickly sent me to the emergency room. I was admitted, and the next morning I had an angioplasty. Doctors found three blockages in my arteries. One artery was 80% blocked, another 90%, and the third 100%. Besides these issues, they found problems with a valve and other small blockages.

Over the next few months, I had three angioplasties resulting in the insertion of four stents in my arteries. During this time, I have relied heavily on God, and He has not let me down. I have also gone to cardiac rehab for my heart, and it was great. I realized this would be beneficial for people with Parkinson's even if they do not have other medical problems. Also, I have found three additional sources of help. The Lancaster County Parkinson's Support Group has been extremely helpful, as have been two internet chat sites. The first site, http://www.wemove.org, is for those with any movement disorder. The second, http://www.parkinsonprofile.com is for those with Parkinson's.

My tremors have continued to worsen. I have also developed problems with balance and memory loss. I began to see double late at night when I was very tired. I sometimes feel the beginnings of "freezing," especially in doorways and tight places. Basically, freezing is not being able to get your feet to move. You essentially get stuck in place for a short while. This has increased and at the same time my "shuffling walk" has gotten worse. All of these problems, particularly the memory loss, have made writing this book especially challenging. But they have also made me more determined to write it now.

My medicines have constantly changed and need to be revised again. I currently take 22 pills a day for PD, heart, arthritis, prostate, and other conditions. I hate meds, and I am concerned that the interaction between medicines will have a long-term impact worse than the diseases themselves. Time will tell. I challenge the doctors each time I go to try and bring down the number of medicines I take daily. But I do realize that the medicines are also what keep me alive.

I have lived a reasonably long life—sixty-eight years so far. I often joke with my family that my job now is to try to stay above ground as long as possible. But even though I joke about it, I take it seriously. My life has been full of hard times and great blessings. And though the hard times continue, God also continues to bless me. I'm trying to stick around to enjoy those blessings as much as possible. And I would like to make a difference in other people's lives. That is what this book is all about. It is my statement, my testimony, that God's grace brings blessing in the midst of difficulty. I wouldn't trade my life for anybody's. With God's help I will finish my journey with class.

Before I close my own story, I would like to share just a little of someone else's. Do you remember Fred Beck? He was Ruth's father and my Sunday school teacher. Of course, he later became my father-in-law. He died in April 1996 at the age of ninety. He had many true stories to tell, and he told them often at family gatherings. There was one that touched my heart more than any other. In 1993, his granddaughter, my daughter, Cheryl gave it a title and put it on paper. I have reproduced it here.

In Over My Head

by Fred V. Beck

As Told to Cheryl L. Miller

For a moment, my head bobbed above the water's surface, and I tried desperately to fill my lungs with air before the swirling rip-tides pulled me under once again. I was growing tired. Too tired to fight much longer against the strong currents threatening to drown me. I didn't even have the strength to call out for help. Even if I could, there was no one around to hear me. I was struggling for my life in this channel...and I was all alone.

It was a beautiful July afternoon in the summer of 1921, a perfect day for a trip to the beach. My father, mother, younger brother Walter and I hopped into the family car and took a ride to Great Kills, a public beach in Staten Island. Almost as soon as the car came to a stop, my brother and I jumped out and took off running, whooping and hollering all the way down the beach. After a while Walter settled down to play in the sand while I decided to go exploring. A short distance down the beach I noticed a group of families crossing a channel of water to a small sandy shoal about one hundred feet away. That looked like an interesting place to explore, so I lit out in that direction. When I reached them, I could see that some of the kids crossing the channel were about my height, and the water only reached their mid-sections. I decided that even though I couldn't swim very well, I would cross the channel too. After all, the water would only come to my waist; it wasn't like I was getting in over my head. I didn't realize, however, that the water was shallow because the tide was out and that my security was only temporary.

I tagged along behind the other kids and their folks and made it easily to the small island. I left the group and took off to start exploring. I was having so much fun that I completely lost track of the time. Soon I realized, much to my dismay, that the sun had sunk considerably lower in the sky. It was getting late. Uh-oh. Father would be angry with me. I'd better head back to the beach on the double. I looked around, trying to find the families I had crossed over with, hoping to follow them back. But no one was around. I looked across to the opposite shore. Not a soul in sight. There weren't even any boats on the horizon. I began to panic. It must be later than I thought; everyone had gone home! Oh boy, Father was going to be furious. I'd better hurry. I knew I was going to have to brave crossing the channel alone, so I started for the water's edge.

HARD TIMES AND GREAT BLESSINGS

Something wasn't right. The water seemed to be moving much more swiftly than before. And it looked a lot higher than I remembered. The tide was coming in—fast. At the time, my eight year old mind didn't comprehend how very dangerous it was to cross the channel during a high tide. All I knew was, high water or not, life wouldn't be worth living anyway if my father had to come and retrieve me. My father was a very hard, strict man, possessing very little patience, and I knew he would not greet my present situation with any degree of sympathy.

I cautiously stepped into the water and started across. The current was swift, and it was hard to make much headway. The hundred feet across the channel seemed like a thousand. The further out I paddled, the deeper the water became, until soon it was completely over my head. I made it about halfway across the channel, and realized I was in serious trouble. The current was merciless, constantly dragging me under, and I couldn't force myself to the surface often enough to get sufficient air. I was drowning. The undertow was overpowering, the shore so far away, and I was exhausted. I would never make it alone. I started going under for the last time.

Suddenly, a pair of strong arms were lifting me out of the water. Coughing and sputtering, I found myself sitting in a small rowboat. Across from me sat a very large man who was quickly rowing us towards the shore. Neither of us spoke. I was still speechless with shock and bewilderment. Where did this guy in the rowboat come from? Only moments before there was no one in sight. Anywhere. And how could he have maneuvered this tiny rowboat to reach me in these riptides? He should have been tossed about like a leaf in the wind. Besides that, how did he even find me? I hadn't even called out for help.

Before I had time to ponder these things further I saw that we had reached the shore. I crawled out of the boat and into the sand. I suddenly realized I hadn't even thanked this man for saving my life. I turned around to do so, but the words fell from my lips as my jaw dropped in disbelief. He was gone. So was the rowboat. I scanned the beach and the horizon. Neither the man nor the rowboat were anywhere in sight.

Seventy-two summers have come and gone since then, and I have never forgotten how the Lord saved my life and the lesson I learned that day. I shall never cease to be grateful that we serve a kind, compassionate God who is always near, watching and protecting us, even at times when we are in way over our heads and feel quite alone. It's a great comfort to know that during difficult times in our lives, when it seems as though we are being dragged down by the eddies and currents of trials and suffering, our precious Savior will not let us drown in sorrow. He will lift us up with His strong, loving arms and set our feet back on solid ground.

EPILOGUE
THE FUTURE

The future is the most elusive of times. We don't know if we even have one or how long it will last or what our quality of life will be. However, I have no doubt that my future will be full of both hard times and great blessings. I know that because I know not only my physical condition and that of my wife but also the certainty of God's great blessings. And I know that Ruth will continue to love me no matter what happens. I know that except God performs a miracle, my Parkinson's will get worse and that the end period of my life won't be pretty. This is a debilitating, progressive disease. I know that Ruth will have to be rechecked often for cancer. But I also know that God's blessings continue to sustain me and my family.

In view of my Parkinson's, heart, arthritis, prostate, and other problems and the large number of pills I have to take, I often think that I don't have a great deal of life left. All of this might make most people look at the future as being bleak at best. However, I would rather look at it as an opportunity to serve God, an opportunity to make a difference.

We all want to know what the future holds. However, we have no way of knowing for sure what is ahead for us. In many ways, the future remains a blank sheet of paper waiting to be written on. But there is something that we can know for sure. We can know that we do not have to go into the future alone. Jesus will go with us. We need to be in the center of His will.

I hope this book will be both a comfort and blessing to you. Most of all, I hope you know Jesus. You have seen how my story began. You have seen something of the trials that have come my way. Knowing Jesus Christ has been the key to all the blessings that have sustained me along the way. If you don't know Him, you can meet Him now. Ask Him for forgiveness and accept His salvation. You will never be sorry. Just remember to give me a wave and a "hey" in heaven.

It is now April, 2008, and this book has been written. One would think this is the end of the story, but it isn't. It is the beginning of the rest of my life. I wanted to slip these comments in before publication and let you in on the latest development. I had been having some double vision problems and went to an eye specialist. He was concerned because the symptoms indicate that I might have myasthenia gravis, a serious muscle disease that affects the eyes. He ordered some tests, and I will be waiting for the results. If I do have this disease, what will the effect be on my future? None! I am determined to serve God and to praise him till the end of my days. Job did, and with God's help so will I. It is my desire to stay in the race through the finish line.

May God richly bless you!

Comments about this book can be sent to:

<u>hardtimes@epix.net</u> *or made on this blog:*

HARD-TIMES-GREAT-BLESSINGS.blogspot.com

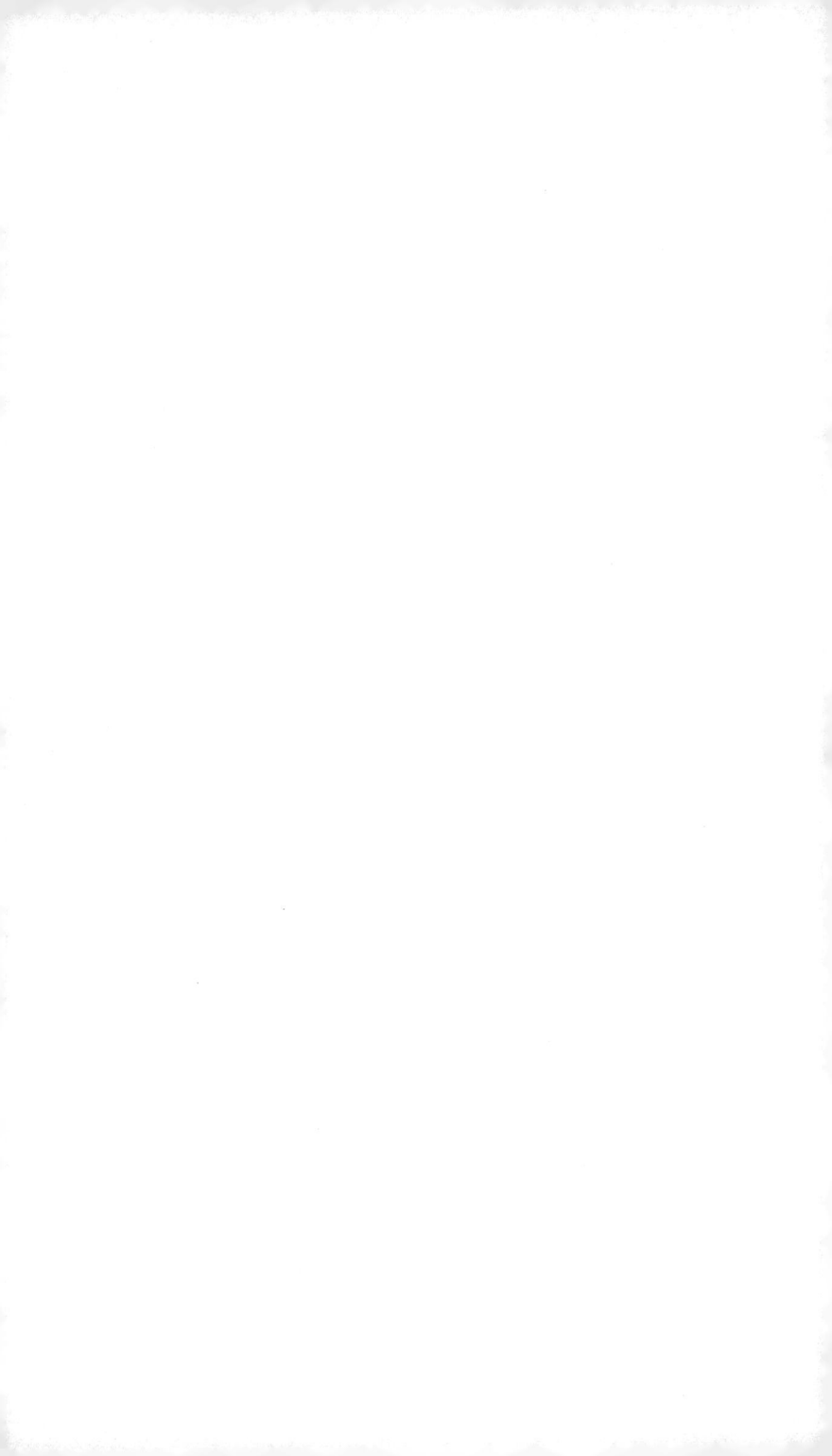

Printed in the United States
204576BV00001B/58-87/P